HISTORICAL PERSPECTIVES ON RURAL MEDICINE

The proceedings of two Witness Seminars held by the
History of Modern Biomedicine Research Group, Queen Mary
University of London, on 29 January 2010 and 3 September 2015

Edited by C Overy and E M Tansey

Volume 61   2017

First published by Queen Mary University of London, 2017

The History of Modern Biomedicine Research Group is funded by the Wellcome Trust, which is a registered charity, no. 210183.

ISBN 978 1 91019 5222

All volumes are freely available online at www.histmodbiomed.org

Please cite as: Overy C, Tansey E M. (eds) (2017) *Historical Perspectives on Rural Medicine. The Proceedings of Two Witness Seminars.* Wellcome Witnesses to Contemporary Medicine, vol. 61. London: Queen Mary University of London.

CONTENTS

WHAT IS A WITNESS SEMINAR?

The Witness Seminar is a specialized form of oral history, where several individuals associated with a particular set of circumstances or events are invited to meet together to discuss, debate, and agree or disagree about their memories. The meeting is recorded, transcribed, and edited for publication.

This format was first devised and used by the Wellcome Trust's History of Twentieth Century Medicine Group in 1993 to address issues associated with the discovery of monoclonal antibodies. We developed this approach after holding a conventional seminar, given by a medical historian, on the discovery of interferon. Many members of the invited audience were scientists or others involved in that work, and the detailed and revealing discussion session afterwards alerted us to the importance of recording 'communal' eyewitness testimonies. We learned that the Institute for Contemporary British History held meetings to examine modern political, diplomatic, and economic history, which they called Witness Seminars, and this seemed a suitable title for us to use also.

The unexpected success of our first Witness Seminar, as assessed by the willingness of the participants to attend, speak frankly, agree and disagree, and also by many requests for its transcript, encouraged us to develop the Witness Seminar model into a full programme, and since then more than 65 meetings have been held and published on a wide array of biomedical topics.[1] These seminars have proved an ideal way to bring together clinicians, scientists, and others interested in contemporary medical history to share their memories. We are not seeking a consensus, but are providing the opportunity to hear an array of voices, many little known, of individuals who were 'there at the time' and thus able to question, ratify, or disagree with others' accounts – a form of open peer-review. The material records of the meeting also create archival sources for present and future use.

The History of Twentieth Century Medicine Group became a part of the Wellcome Trust's Centre for the History of Medicine at UCL in October 2000 and remained so until September 2010. It has been part of the School of History, Queen Mary University of London, since October 2010, as the History of Modern Biomedicine Research Group, which the Wellcome Trust

---

[1] See pages 191–7 for a full list of Witness Seminars held, details of the published volumes and other related publications.

funds principally under a Strategic Award entitled 'The Makers of Modern Biomedicine'. The Witness Seminar format continues to be a major part of that programme, although now the subjects are largely focused on areas of strategic importance to the Wellcome Trust, including the neurosciences, clinical genetics, and medical technology.[2]

Once an appropriate topic has been agreed, usually after discussion with a specialist adviser, suitable participants are identified and invited. As the organization of the Seminar progresses and the participants' list is compiled, a flexible outline plan for the meeting is devised, with assistance from the meeting's designated chairman/moderator. Each participant is sent an attendance list and a copy of this programme before the meeting. Seminars last for about four hours; occasionally full-day meetings have been held. After each meeting the raw transcript is sent to every participant, each of whom is asked to check his or her own contribution and to provide brief biographical details for an appendix. The editors incorporate participants' minor corrections and turn the transcript into readable text, with footnotes, appendices, and a bibliography. Extensive research and liaison with the participants is conducted to produce the final script, which is then sent to every contributor for approval and to assign copyright to the Wellcome Trust. Copies of the original, and edited, transcripts and additional correspondence generated by the editorial process are all deposited with the records of each meeting in the Wellcome Library, London (archival reference GC/253) and are available for study.

For all our volumes, we hope that, even if the precise details of the more technical sections are not clear to the non-specialist, the sense and significance of the events will be understandable to all readers. Our aim is that the volumes inform those with a general interest in the history of modern medicine and medical science; provide historians with new insights, fresh material for study, and further themes for research; and emphasize to the participants that their own working lives are of proper and necessary concern to historians.

---

[2]   See our group's website at www.histmodbiomed.org

ACKNOWLEDGEMENTS

A Witness Seminar on rural medicine was suggested in 2009 by Professor Roger Strasser and Professor John Hamilton, and planned for later that year. Transport difficulties meant the original meeting was postponed, and eventually a smaller, more focused seminar than was originally intended was held in January 2010. This served as a useful introduction to the topic, and we envisioned holding an additional, more substantial, meeting to add more comprehensive and international dimensions to the published proceedings. Administrative changes and physical relocations delayed further organization until mid-2013, at which point the plan was resurrected, with the additional help of Professor Geoffrey Hudson, medical historian at Northern Ontario School of Medicine. To overcome the logistics of arranging such an international discussion it was decided to hold the second meeting with the majority of overseas participants contributing via video links; this was held in September 2015. We are very grateful to Roger Strasser, John Hamilton, Geoffrey Hudson, and also Dr John Wynn-Jones for their help in planning these meetings, and to Roger and Professor Sir Denis Pereira Gray for chairing the Witness Seminars.

The initial intention was to meld the proceedings of the two meetings into one published account. However, after reviewing both transcripts, it became apparent to the editors that the two volumes could not only be read independently but they also complemented each other. Thus we are publishing them together but organized in reverse order to that in which they were held. We thank Geoffrey Hudson for writing an introduction that includes both meetings.

Our thanks also goes to the participants for providing many of the images used, and to the Wellcome Library, London, for permission to use photographs taken at the meeting. As with all our meetings, we depend a great deal on Wellcome Trust staff to ensure their smooth running: Audiovisual, Catering, Reception, Security, and Wellcome Images. We are also grateful to Mr Akio Morishima for the design and production of this volume; the indexer Ms Cath Topliff; Mrs Sarah Beanland and Ms Fiona Plowman for proofreading; Ms Dee Briston and Mrs Debra Gee for transcribing the seminars; and Mrs Wendy Kutner, Mrs Lois Reynolds, and Dr Carole Reeves, who assisted in the organization and running of the meetings as did Mr Adam Wilkinson who also managed the complex video link arrangements of the second meeting. Finally, we thank the Wellcome Trust for supporting this programme.

Tilli Tansey and Caroline Overy
School of History, Queen Mary University of London

ILLUSTRATIONS AND CREDITS*

* Unless otherwise stated, all photographs were taken by David Bishop, Wellcome Trust, and reproduced courtesy of the Wellcome Library, London. Photographs from the 2010 Witness Seminar (Figures 28–36) were taken by a member of the History of Twentieth Century Medicine Group.

ABBREVIATIONS

ACRRM	Australian College of Rural and Remote Medicine
AIDA	Australian Indigenous Doctors Association
AMA	Australian Medical Association
AMC	Australian Medical Council
BASICS	British Association of Immediate Care Systems
BMA	British Medical Association
CBL	case-based learning
COPD	chronic obstructive pulmonary disease
CPD	continuing professional development
EBM	evidence-based medicine
EURIPA	European Rural and Isolated Practitioners Association
GMC	General Medical Council
ICOH	International Commission on Occupational Health
JCU	James Cook University
KoHOM	Croatian Family Physicians Coordination
PA	Physician Assistant
PBL	problem-based learning
RARARI	Remote and Rural Areas Resource Initiative
RARM	Remote and Rural Medicine
RCOG	Royal College of Obstetricians and Gynaecologists
RHAANZ	Rural Health Alliance Aotearoa New Zealand
RCGP	Royal College of General Practitioners
RuDASA	Rural Doctors Association of Southern Africa
RUSC	Rural Undergraduate Steering Committee

THET	Tropical Health & Education Trust
Wits	Witwatersrand, University,
WONCA	World Organization of National Colleges, Academies and Academic Associations of General Practitioners/Family Physicians; shortened to World Organization of Family Doctors

INTRODUCTION

'… the goal of health for our rural people … is not an eight-lane superhighway, it's a wandering road through the bush with many unexpected challenges along the way …. Rural practice still faces those challenges but we have a whole cadre of people now involved in rural practice as rural doctors, and hopefully we'll take this forward because I do think it is a need that still requires high profile leadership to maintain the focus on providing health to the people in communities, which is what people around here have been working on all this time. So an exciting time period but it will remain a challenge ….'

Dr James Rourke[1]

I was delighted to accept the invitation to write this introduction. I teach History of Medicine in the Northern Ontario School of Medicine, a school recently created (charter class 2005) to provide rural and remote medical education. Working in this medical school can resemble life in a small town, with each of us faculty members wearing several hats simultaneously. In my case this has included coordinating a seven-week module – unique in the world – which requires all first-year students to go into indigenous communities across the vast area of Northern Ontario for an immersion educational experience.[2] Co-ordinating this challenging module has been a joy and privilege. Another component of the job, like that of historians in medical schools elsewhere, concerns the medical school – the institution itself. In this capacity, for example, I helped to edit a book chronicling the efforts to create the medical school.[3] I also, as Roger Strasser comments below, recommended a Witness Seminar for this international discussion of the development of rural medicine. In this introduction, I will briefly summarize the discussion organized by the themes used in the Seminar, and then comment on potential areas for further consideration and research.

Impact of specialization

Specialism was seen as well established by the 1970s, to varying degrees depending on locale. Australia, for example, was seeing students going into specialist rather than general practice by that point in time. The same pattern, with slightly different time scales was apparent elsewhere. The long-term trend was seen to

---

[1] See page 79.

[2] Hudson and Maar (2014).

[3] Tesson *et al.* (eds) (2009).

have created a hierarchy, with GPs/family practitioners lower down the scale than urban specialists, and rural doctors even lower down. The pharmaceutical companies played a part, with funding going to specialists; rural practitioners were not deemed a group that could do appropriate studies. Another element of specialization was the development of large urban hospitals, with rural hospitals closed in many locations (e.g. Norway). It led to centralization of services, which was challenging for those practising in rural areas, and also led to sub-specialist development. Growing specialization raised patient expectations for complete equity in health services which, were not always realistic. Guidelines for practice were developed in some places that were simply unworkable in rural areas.

The response by rural practitioners was seen as multifaceted: rural practice specialities were created (e.g. UK); there were moves to have smaller, rural hospitals set up, to re-ruralize health care (e.g. Tasmania); new medical schools were established with a rural and remote mission; and rural curriculum was developed for pre-existing schools, which was sometimes contentious for some traditional medical schools (e.g. Canada).[4]

There were continued challenges. Rural health educators in medical schools in some locales were still facing opposition from hospital-based specialists. The hope was expressed that although the period 1970–2000 saw a swing from generalized to sub-specialization, other changes had occurred that might well lead to an appropriate balance over time. Part of this hope rested on changes in areas such as technology. Rural practitioners now had access and support from specialists in many remote and rural places in which it had previously been unavailable. It was also stated that conditions had improved such that in many places most rural practitioners were enjoying being rural practitioners. This was deemed beneficial for recruitment.

Nature of generalism and its relationship to rural medicine

The history of generalism is, of course, related closely to the impact of specialism. In many parts of the world generalism was seen as continuing well into the latter part of the twentieth century. This was particularly the case in the rural setting. Participants commented on aspects of earlier twentieth-century developments including awareness that the general practitioner model of northern Scotland was influential in the development of the NHS of 1948;[5] sometimes rural innovations

---

[4] See page 41.

[5] See pages 77 and 87–9.

in general practice influenced the cities. The separation of general practice from hospital practice in the UK resulted in significant restrictions on admitting rights for generalists in the larger hospitals. New and different divisions were created between specialists and generalists, as with other health professions. In some countries urban generalists limited their practice in ways that contrasted with the complexity of practice required in remote and rural areas.

The WONCA (World Organization of Family Doctors) Working Party on Rural Practice defined rural practitioners as extended generalists.[6] Such physicians were to provide a wider range of services, at a higher level of clinical responsibility. There is relative professional isolation, which is mitigated by other developments such as technologically facilitated communication. Part of the job is dealing with emergencies, and there is a community public health dimension. There is now an important role in medical education for rural general practice teaching in part because it teaches a wide range of treatments and communication skills.

Professional identity and status

The 1980s and 1990s were a particularly important time for the reinvigoration of professional identity by rural doctors via their own support networks, nationally and internationally. They developed common goals and understandings on a wide array of related matters.

There was acknowledgement that rural practitioners were and are informed of their own heritage as rural doctors both through viewing artwork, and reading rural doctor biographies and memoirs.[7] They had heard, and passed on, the tales of remarkable country doctors, who survived hardship to provide good care. Several spoke of their own experience in remote practice and its challenges. Some rural practitioners in countries like Canada and Australia practise in bush and forest, providing services to indigenous populations that have their own health care understandings and traditions. Participants spoke of taking pride in knowing their patients and their needs in a way that differs significantly from urban practitioners. They also commented on the importance of rural medicine in preserving rural identity and power for communities.[8] The value of a good understanding of their own history was discussed, not only in and of itself, but also for effective professional engagement with the public and government.

---

[6] See page 95.

[7] See pages 78 and 105.

[8] See pages 111–12.

However, there was a need for caution with respect to claiming disadvantage to justify demands for support, while at the same time trying to encourage future practitioners to come on board.

Impact of technological developments (transportation and communication)

As early as the 1912 Report of the (Scottish) Highlands and Islands Medical Service Committee (the Dewar Report), suggestions were made for better use of telephones and the internal combustion engine (e.g. horseless ambulances) to improve rural health care. For the period of focus (1970–2000) mention was made of the importance of short wave radio in the 1970s and 1980s (e.g. journal clubs),[9] as well as the slightly later use of the fax machine and teleconference, with the creation of rural physician networks, the sharing of information and support, and continuing education.

Once computers were available rural doctors were early users, creating patient registers and later using email to get in touch with each other for clinical support. As the internet developed further the use of information technology expanded significantly, with videoconferences possible by the late 1990s – and it is so appropriate that such technology was employed for this Witness Seminar!

Telemedicine began in earnest in many locations, such as Newfoundland, with an early satellite project developed to connect rural practitioners, including access to specialist advice and support.[10] This made it possible for many patients to stay and receive care in their own communities. As the years passed telemedicine expanded to include tele-pharmacy, point of care ECG, ultrasound and more besides. Telemedicine, combined with transportation improvements, (ambulances, including helicopters) made it possible to better identify, and then relatively quickly transport, the patients that really did need to go to major centres.

Technology also made new forms of rural medical research possible (e.g. research funded by the European Space Agency into the risk of Lyme disease, using a mobile phone app),[11] and the internet improved the health literacy of patients, thereby improving patient communication.

---

[9] See page 54.

[10] See page 66.

[11] See page 34.

There had been challenges, and there are ongoing problems. Governments fell in and out of love with new technologies, establishing pilot projects and then failing to continue them (e.g. telemedicine in mid-Wales and Shropshire in the 1990s).[12] Sometimes those in government misunderstand the importance and necessity of rural practitioners, thinking that telemedicine could replace rather than support them. In some cases telehealth was imposed in problematic ways rather than developed from the bottom up. In some places, broadband internet is still not available in a consistent way (e.g. New Zealand, mountainous areas of the UK).[13] And there was worry that the more recent sophistication of the internet could be challenging, with physicians going online for information rather than engaging in and with their rural networks.

In sum, several participants commented that technology had improved the capacity and power of rural practitioners, and by doing so improved their ability to provide better health care.

National and international networks and organizations

Overall, the networks and organizations created in the period were seen as re-imagining and reinforcing the professional identity of the rural physician, the key period identified being the late 1980s and 1990s. Led by Australia and rural practitioners in other countries, rural physicians were brought together globally. Participants identified their involvement in the World Health Organization and an eventual set of guidelines in 2010 as mainstreaming their issues internationally, including increasing access to health workers in remote and rural areas via retention and other measures.[14]

In Australia, a conference in 1978, 'Country Towns, Country Doctors', helped to raise expectations that were not initially fulfilled.[15] Rural doctors created very influential rural physician organizations (training and practice) in the late 1980s and 1990s, including the Rural Doctors Association and the College of Rural and Remote Medicine. In other countries there were other developments (e.g. Belgrade conference on Rural Health; Remote Practitioners' Association in Scotland; and Association of Rural Surgeons in India). UK practitioners,

---

[12] See page 62.

[13] See pages 63–4 and 65.

[14] World Health Organization (2010).

[15] See pages 145–6.

experiencing some challenges, pointed to examples from other countries such as Australia as inspirational and useful.

Globally the WONCA Working Party on Rural Practice (established in 1992) and other organizations brought rural practitioners together at key conferences internationally (e.g. Hong Kong in 1995).[16] Rural physicians found they had more in common with each other than colleagues in urban areas.

Relationship to other health professions

GPs, nurses, and other health care providers worked together on the front lines to provide secure access for patients in small communities. They learned to join forces with all the effort and challenges that entails – communication, mutual encouragement, and support, for example, on one occasion, switching places with an ambulance driver in outback Australia.[17] Usually the team is led by a physician, although not always – context is important: a midwife could lead a maternity unit if a consultant was available nearby.[18] Participants discussed the benefits of having a generalist physician do the triage.

In many countries para-professional community health workers are of crucial importance. Medical assistants, clinical officers, village health workers and others provided valuable services such as vaccination and much more besides, throughout Africa as well as other countries, such as Iran. These were experienced workers, who in some places worked more closely and successfully with physicians than others.

As with telehealth development, there were erratic problems with government funding with respect to inter-professional education (e.g. Canada); some governments promise to provide nurse practitioners and physician assistants but then either do not deliver or deliver them in inappropriate ways (e.g. centrally planned).

Several participants mentioned that other health care providers in some locales experience the same difficulties as physicians: the necessity of providing a relatively wide range of service at a high level in professional isolation. Remote nursing station personnel are subject to burnout much like physicians.[19]

---

[16] Couper *et al.* (2015).

[17] See page 107.

[18] See pages 139–40.

[19] See page 108.

Urban-rural relationship and divide

With respect to the urban-rural relationship and divide, and the development of rural medicine, there has been a long-term urban transition, with a majority of the world's population inhabiting urban areas by 2009.[20] Rural physicians for decades had been dealing with a rural/urban divide in terms of hospital service capabilities, and attitudes, with the specialist in the urban hospital and the rural general practitioner being seen by some urban types as polar opposites in terms of both standards and career desirability. The latter prejudices had negatively impacted student recruitment, resulting in rural doctor shortages in some countries. Specific resource allocation problems were cited, with government attitudes and initiatives favouring centralization in urban areas.

It was observed that rural patients consistently wanted to be cared for in their rural areas. The hospital in the urban area was perceived to be de-personalizing, while the cottage hospital was home.[21]

The response on the part of rural doctors and some governments over the years has been multifaceted, with the establishment of rural practice networks (e.g. New Zealand) and rural medicine as a distinct discipline responsive to the needs of the community. Some countries and medical schools had required rural training, increased rural practitioner salaries (e.g. Thailand), and/or recruited future physicians from the rural areas (e.g. Nigeria). Many of these strategies have been successful.

There was some discussion of the success of rural practitioners 'pulling up the drawbridge' in 1990s Australia as a tactic to in part place emphasis on skill development in rural areas.[22] Some participants commented on the benefit of an alliance with those practising in pockets of post-industrialization, which in some ways resembled rural areas in terms of health inequities and isolation.

Participants from some countries pointed out that in their locales more needed to be done, with Bosnia, for example, still favouring urban doctors such that their rural counterparts had to do a significant portion of work without compensation. The UK was being cited as a place focused on metropolitan concerns, with unintended negative consequences with regard to more recent NHS policy initiatives.

---

[20] See pages 58 and 97.

[21] See page 116.

[22] See page 59.

Social accountability and equity

There were comments about the long-term development of equity and social accountability concerns related to rural health. The Dewar Report of 1912 declared that rural people have a right to medical and midwifery services. Discussion also included developments in South Africa prior to the Nationalists coming to power in 1948, with respect to community-orientated primary care, and how this orientation had been reinstituted more recently. Participants emphasized that social accountability means having a relationship with the communities, listening to them and responding with services that corresponded to their articulated needs. This made the rural practitioner distinct from the urban practitioner the latter of whom might live in one place but practise in another. It was commented that it was crucial to avoid reductionism in social accountability – to focus only on the economic efficiency of services.[23] Several participants mentioned that part of the role of the rural practitioner is to research access and other issues related to rural practice (e.g. cancer patients in rural Scotland).

In comments on rural and remote medical education participants linked it to social accountability and equity. There was the example of northern Norway and Dr Peter Hjort and colleagues who created the medical school at the University of Tromsø, to serve the north, an underprivileged area prior to 1970. Students spend the fifth year in rural areas with rural practitioners, and in local hospitals.[24] James Cook University's medical school in Australia was founded to train future physicians to serve rural and Aboriginal patients and communities. It was emphasized that students are sent to communities rather than practices. Others commented that students need to learn in, and from, the communities, and in some cases from subgroups of disadvantaged (e.g. ex-convicts). Several participants raised occupational health as an example of social accountability in action for rural practitioners. Living in a community means responding to and investigating occupational health problems, for example James Douglas' role in investigating aquaculture, fish farming, and asthma.[25] Participants commented on mining, forestry, manufacturing, and occupational diseases (e.g. aluminium factory and COPD (chronic obstructive pulmonary disease)).

---

[23] See page 74.

[24] See page 20.

[25] See page 34.

Despite the challenges related to the social accountability role – slur of 'the barefoot doctor'[26] – the status of the rural practitioner is high in the communities. With the recent move of the doctor's office out of the home in most places one might think this would negatively affect the connection with the community, however the sense of social responsibility very much remains, for example, rural practitioners' actions on behalf of the community during the foot and mouth outbreak in the UK in 2001.[27] There was acknowledgement of the challenge of war and migration in many parts of the world (e.g. Balkans) over the period, on health care, including rural health care. In the UK, more recent NHS centralization was perceived to be threatening their connection with their patients.

Gender

There was a masculine element to the old image of the super rural physician capable of doing anything.[28] It was a macho image. This manifested itself not only in terms of the place of the male practitioner's wife but increasingly the female rural doctor. Indeed, since the 1970s there were many more women in medicine, and a need to attract them to rural practice.

Studies that focused particularly on issues preventing female practitioners going into, or feeling comfortable in, rural areas,[29] showed that what was needed was further engagement with female future physicians and graduates in deciding how to deal with issues related to rural practice, including their participation in it.

In some areas there has been a more recent push to respond to violence against women in rural areas in terms of both medical curriculum and practice. This included an ongoing relationship with women's shelters in order to better take care of the victims of domestic violence.[30]

With the current generation's expressed concerns for greater work–life balance, there was an attraction to specialist rather than generalist medicine in some locales, which was seen by some as a challenge.

---

[26] See pages 39 and 45.

[27] See page 115.

[28] See page 70.

[29] Commonwealth Department of Human Services and Health (1994). See also WONCA Working Party on Rural Practice (2003).

[30] See pages 32 and 73.

Families

The connection of home and doctor's office put stresses and strains upon the family, with the entire family being, in one sense, rural practitioners, and the fishbowl effect – with everyone watching and commenting on family activities.[31] This led to ever-ringing door bells and losing pieces of family property to light-fingered patients, but also to the existence of respect of local people for the physician and family.[32] To help deal with the family strain, in some places (Australia) rural networks were created for women and families,[33] although the advent of policy changes in other locales (New Zealand) had put pressure on those networks.[34] The history of this work–life balance strain has had an effect on the latest generation, with an acknowledged attractiveness of specialist practice, as compared to generalist rural practice, for current young female future physicians with children.

Sustainability (education, financial, personal, and professional supports)

Finally we come to sustainability: the future. This theme was of great concern and one of the most discussed themes overall. Participants addressed personal and professional support problems, and lessons learned. The realities of living in remote and rural areas among small populations were discussed – long distances, difficult terrain, communication and transport problems, limited resources, professional isolation, and burnout. Solutions included making the most of what is available: the new technologies; access to and support from appropriate specialists; the creation of health care teams; being embedded in the community and growing comfortable with being in the fishbowl. A crucial support identified is the rural population itself – comfortable that their health needs are serviced.

Medical education in the sustainability of rural practice was seen as critically important. Recruitment and subsequent education challenges and solutions were highlighted. It had been found in several medical schools that recruiting from the rural and remote populations produced long-term success with respect to students later practising in rural and remote areas. It was seen that

---

[31] See pages 70 and 152.

[32] See page 153.

[33] See page 26.

[34] See page 74.

during training, students needed to receive positive reinforcement – good patient outcomes – rather than negative examples about rural medicine. Small group case scenarios for students needed to be situated in rural and remote communities and practice. Students needed to be sent out to rural communities to learn to relate to the communities and to learn how to practise there. Learning in context, including immersion, was key, with longitudinal rural clerkships as an important component. Detailed, careful, assessment of the students was vital. Some schools had been more successful than others but lessons were being shared actively. Good examples of rural and remote health care recruitment, education and retention were discussed (e.g. northern Norway).[35]

Participants recognized that students needed to understand that rural generalist practice training would enhance their education and practice no matter what kind of practice they would eventually end up in. Schools needed to develop a philosophy that would instil pride on the part of students in the school, rural practice, and their future role.

The support (or lack thereof) by government was identified as being very influential in the sustainability of rural medicine. Australia had struggled successfully earlier on (e.g. 1980s rural practice compensation issues), and struggles with government were particularly identified at length by UK participants. They were greatly concerned with the adverse effect of the centralization direction of government, rigidity of work time rules, lack of response to rural practitioners' concerns, rural health underfunding, and recruitment difficulties. Some of these concerns were echoed by others from other jurisdictions (e.g. Bosnia).

What gave some hope was the view that governments should recognize that the most efficient and cost-effective health service is comprehensive primary healthcare. With respect to a global perspective, there were certain countries in which rural practice sustainability was in hand (Australia, Canada, USA, South Africa, Norway were cited); these provided inspirational examples for others in their ongoing struggles.

As per James Rourke's quote at the beginning of this introduction, leadership was acknowledged as being key to sustaining rural medical practice and education over the long term and into the future.

---

[35] See pages 56–7.

Conclusion

The Witness Seminar as a form of focus group consideration of an historical theme is useful in many ways. It creates, for example, a source for discussion and action on the part of scholars, pointing to fruitful areas for further research. In this review of the themes I have, on occasion, mentioned the agency and voice of patients in the rural areas. It is clear that they (and the rural communities) animate and inspire the physician practitioners, scientists, and educators who gathered for this Witness Seminar. Certainly more research could be done to draw on the patient and community voice and experience, and this would greatly add to our appreciation of relevant changes and continuities over the period.

As Tilli Tansey remarked, the voice of other health practitioners (and I would add para-professionals) would enrich our understanding of this important aspect of the history of medicine.[36] They would tell us more about the history of the development and nature of the health care team.

I want to know more about the distinctive aspects of rural and remote medical practice, as well as the tension between social accountability and equity, for practitioners and educators. With respect to the latter, I concluded in a chapter on social accountability and medical education that communities differ, one from another, on what they want – hard decisions need to be made – and what communities want does not always lead to equitable outcomes for all community members.[37]

I found the discussion of historical events and their impact on the development of rural medicine tantalizingly brief *and* significant – the pre 1970s developments in medicine education (Flexner), the impact of colonialism and its formal end and/or evolution in several countries, the wind down of the communist experiment in so many parts of the world, the increase in urbanization (with the 2009 tipping point mentioned above), the development of post-industrialization in many Western cities in the advent of globalization, and last but not least, generational changes in student and practitioner attitudes towards work–life balance. More could and should be done to analyse and explain the impact of these events and processes for rural medicine and health.

---

[36] See page 151.

[37] Hudson and Hunt (2009).

As someone who comes from the rural periphery of Canada, and teaches in a remote and rural medical school, I found this Seminar fascinating and useful. Indeed, while writing this introduction I found myself using what I had learned from this Witness Seminar to frame my discussion with faculty colleagues about curriculum matters under current consideration. I trust that the reader will draw inspiration and learn lessons from the discussion of these internationally diverse leaders in rural and remote medical practice and education.

Professor Geoffrey Hudson

Northern Ontario School of Medicine
(Faculty of Medicine, Lakehead and
Laurentian Universities, Canada)

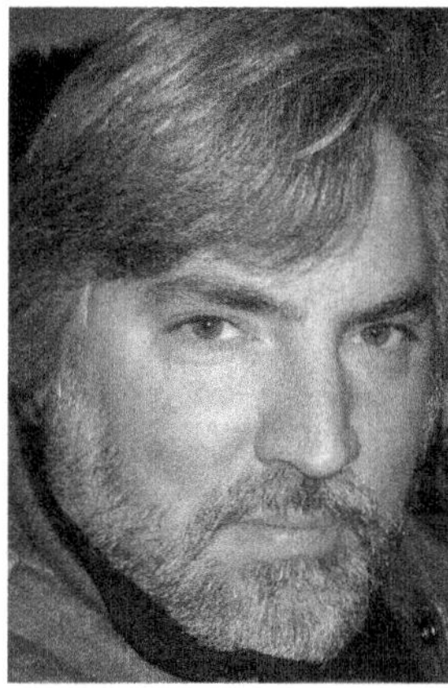

Figure A

HISTORICAL PERSPECTIVES ON RURAL MEDICINE. THE PROCEEDINGS OF TWO WITNESS SEMINARS

Edited by C Overy and E M Tansey

THE DEVELOPMENT OF RURAL MEDICINE c.1970–c.2000

The transcript of a Witness Seminar held by the History of Modern Biomedicine Research Group, Queen Mary University of London, on 3 September 2015

THE DEVELOPMENT OF RURAL MEDICINE c.1970–c.2000

Participants*

Attending in the Wellcome Building

Dr James Douglas
Professor Richard Hays
Professor James Rourke

Professor Roger Strasser (Chair)
Professor Sarah Strasser
Professor Tilli Tansey (Convenor)

Attending via video link

Professor Ivar Aaraas (Norway)
Professor Petar Bulat (Serbia)
Professor Bruce Chater (Australia)
Professor Ian Couper (South Africa)
Professor John Hamilton (Australia)
Professor Victor Inem (Nigeria)
Dr Oleg Kravtchenko (Norway)

Dr Tanja Pekez-Pavlisko (Croatia)
Professor Maja Račić (Bosnia and
    Herzegovina)
Ms Jane Randall-Smith (Wales)
Dr Jo Scott-Jones (New Zealand)
Dr John Wynn-Jones (Wales)

Apologies include: Dr Jose Abuin (Spain), Dr Robert Bowman (USA),
Dr John Gillies (Scotland), Dr Tom Norris (USA), Dr Agnes Simek (Hungary),
Dr Leonardo Targa (Brazil), Dr Ndifreke Udonwa (Nigeria)

* Biographical notes on the participants are located at the end of the volume

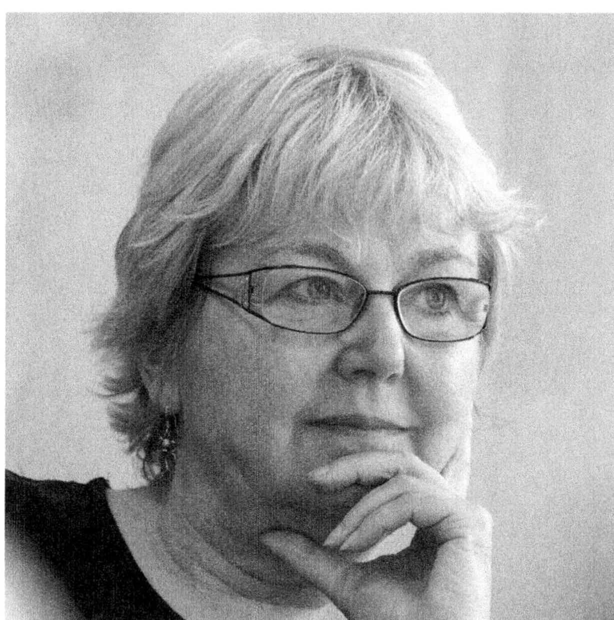

Figure 1: Professor Tilli Tansey

Professor Tilli Tansey: Hello everyone. Good afternoon and good evening, and indeed even good morning depending where you are in the world. This is quite a big experiment for us so please bear with us.[1] We've never done anything like this before. We hold these Witness Seminars as ways of trying to get to people who were involved in various discoveries or debates, to look at the transition of the past 30–40 years, what really happened, what were the drivers, what went wrong, what happened in a particular field? The idea of holding a Witness Seminar on rural medicine came initially from Roger Strasser and John Hamilton about seven or eight years ago now. We held a small meeting in 2010 and, for some time, Roger and I have been talking about trying to have a larger meeting and we very much hope that this is going to be that meeting. What we want to hear about are your own personal experiences over the period from about 1970–2000, the development of rural medicine in your particular areas, and the development of rural medicine education. The format is going to be different and perhaps a little difficult and we're all learning today. I think you are all much more familiar with this technology than we are, so please bear with us. The whole meeting will be recorded, transcribed, and edited for publication in conjunction with that first meeting. So, without further ado, I'm going to hand over to Roger to say a little bit more.

---

[1] This was the first Witness Seminar in which the majority of the participants contributed via a video link.

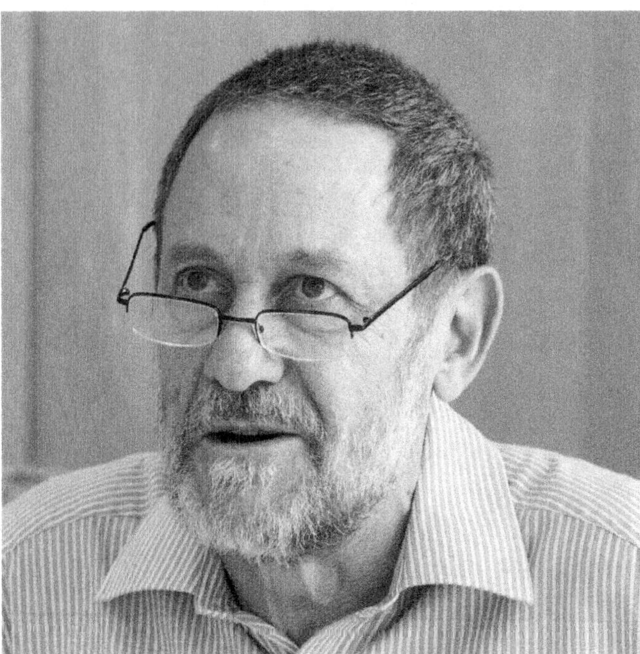

Figure 2: Professor Roger Strasser

Professor Roger Strasser: Well, thank you very much, Tilli, and I would like to welcome you all to this very, very special event. As Tilli has said, it really is a first of its kind for the Witness Seminars in the history of medicine and, I guess, a first of its kind for us in rural medicine as well. I thank you all for your participation, particularly those who have joined us in the middle of the night and will have the staying power for this discussion over four hours. I think that's fantastic. As Tilli said, the genesis of having this Witness Seminar actually goes back to 2005, when I was invited to speak at an academic farewell for John Hamilton, and it's wonderful to have you with us today, John.[2] But back in 2005, John was just finishing a five-year involvement at Durham University in the north of England. That was a new medical school in the north of England, and that's when I discovered that John had been involved in starting four new medical schools on four continents in four different decades, and it seemed to me, well, that kind of experience ought to be documented. So I consulted with the historian of medicine at Northern Ontario School of Medicine, Geoff Hudson, and he recommended connecting with Tilli and then the rest took its course as Tilli has described. Of course, I knew John as the Dean of Medicine at

---

[2] A two-day international conference 'Medical Education: Thinking Globally, Acting Locally' was arranged at the University of Durham in June 2005 to celebrate the career of Professor John Hamilton.

University of Newcastle in Australia and the chair of the Rural Undergraduate Steering Committee and so John certainly, as you'll hear, had involvement in the development of rural medicine in Australia and many other countries as well.

We did actually have a mini Witness Seminar here in London in January of 2010.[3] That was probably more of a focus on rural medicine in the UK, Scotland and England and Wales, and we hope to publish the two meetings together. We did then talk about having further mini seminars in other parts of the world and maybe a big, big Witness Seminar here in London. Last year, as we were chewing over how we were going to do this, suddenly the light went on. Part of the history of rural medicine is the conference call – the electronic communications that allow rural doctors to connect with each other and get organized and so that was a major element. So we thought: 'Well, let's do this Witness Seminar as a conference call', and we are finally, in September of 2015, here for this Witness Seminar. So it is breaking new ground, it's the first one if its kind in terms of an international multi-site conference call and it's the first one that has more of an international dimension and less a history of medicine in the twentieth century with a UK focus. So thank you again for all your participation today. The one-page outline, in case you're wondering where that came from, again I want to acknowledge Geoff Hudson, the historian of medicine at the Northern Ontario School of Medicine. He interviewed me on two different occasions and distilled the key themes really from those interviews, which then were further distilled and became the outline for the programme (Table 1).

When we did the mini Witness Seminar we did it in two parts. We focused on practice for the first part and then education in the second. But as we reflected on that, and working with Geoff, it seemed to make more sense to actually recognize that practice and education are so intertwined. So for this Witness Seminar we're going to explore the genesis and the development of rural medicine with the practice and education dimensions really combined as we go through. I will start off by asking you each to introduce yourself and the perspective that you bring to this Witness Seminar. We need this to be brief enough that we don't spend the whole four hours just introducing ourselves, but long enough that there's a sense not only for ourselves but for those who read the published record in the future to have a sense of who you are and what you're bringing to this conversation. Then I'm going to be encouraging very much an interactive discussion, working through the topics as listed, and I'll be moderating the conversation. I'm going to

---

[3] The Witness Seminar 'The History of Rural Medicine and Rural Medical Education' was held in January 2010, page 83 onwards.

- Impact of specialization
- Nature of generalism and its relationship to rural medicine practice
- Professional identity and status
- Impact of technological developments (transportation and communication)
- National and international networks and organizations
- Relationship to other health professions
- Urban–rural relationship and divide
- Social accountability and equity
- Gender
- Families
- Sustainability (education, financial, personal, and professional supports)

Table 1: Outline programme for the Witness Seminar on
'The Development of Rural Medicine c.1970–c.2000'

encourage all of you to contribute, but also discourage anyone from dominating. It's going to be important that we get the mix of perspectives from individuals around the world. I'll start the ball rolling by introducing myself.

My name is Roger Strasser. My background is as a rural general practitioner or family doctor in Australia, and with quite an academic involvement over the years. I guess my journey in this regard started in 1981 when I came to the UK to undertake some further training, preparing to be a rural doctor and training in surgery and anaesthesia. That's actually where I met Sarah, and that led to our lifelong relationship since then. Then in 1983 I took the opportunity to go to Canada and undertake some academic training with the University of Western Ontario and Ian McWhinney at the Department of Family Medicine there.[4] I went back to Australia into rural practice in a town called Moe and then got involved in various academic activities associated with Monash University, which is in Melbourne, a big city, but Moe has a population of about 17,000, two hours from Melbourne. I got involved with Monash and then the opportunity came in 1992 to be involved in establishing a rural health academic unit, which started off as the Centre for Rural Health for Monash University and then evolved into a School of Rural Health, a rural branch of the Metropolitan Medical School.[5] By the time I left in 2002 the school had four

---

[4] Dr Ian Renwick McWhinney (1926–2012) was an English general practitioner and academic, known as the 'Father of Family Medicine' for his work in creating a family medicine programme at the University of Western Ontario, and holding the first chair in family medicine in Canada. See Kermode-Scott (2012).

[5] For a history of the Monash University School of Rural Health, see Clough (ed.) (2012).

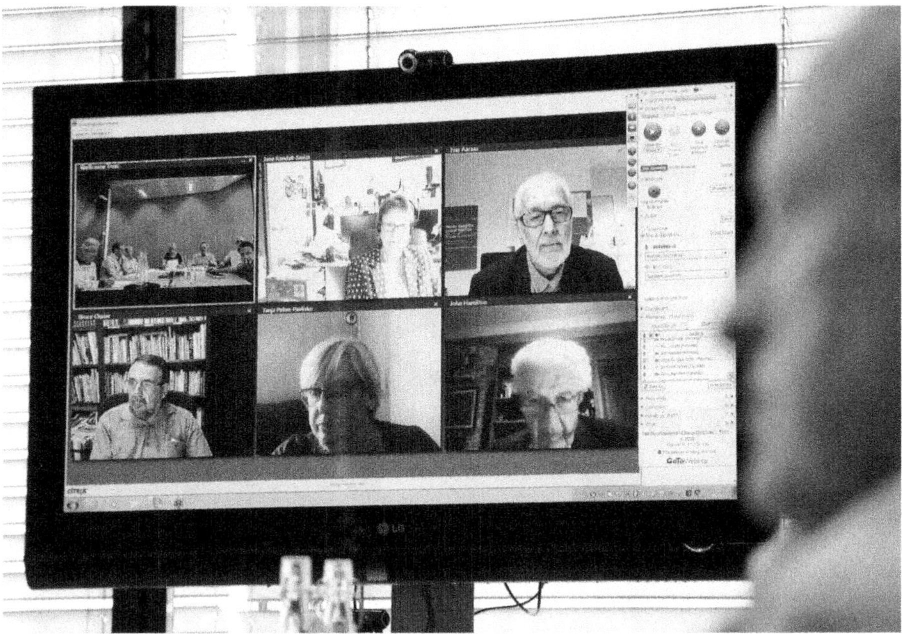

Figure 3: Witness Seminar screen. Clockwise from top left: Conference Room, the
Wellcome Trust; Ms Jane Randall-Smith (Wales); Professor Ivar Aaraas (Norway);
Professor John Hamilton (Australia); Dr Tanja Pekez-Pavlisko (Croatia);
Professor Bruce Chater (Australia)

main sites and a network of other teaching and research sites across quite a large
rural area in the state of Victoria in Australia. Then in 2002, the opportunity
came to move back to Canada and to be involved in establishing a full medical
school that was multi-site and rural-based.

I became involved in starting the Northern Ontario School of Medicine, which
had its official opening in 2005, and so in 2015 we're celebrating our tenth
anniversary.[6] I guess my other relevant background to this discussion today is
that in 1992 I was attending the WONCA (World Organization of Family
Doctors)[7] World Conference, and there were quite a few rural doctors there
and we got talking. One thing led to another and that was the beginning of

---

[6] For a history of the Northern Ontario School of Medicine, see Tesson *et al.* (eds) (2009).

[7] WONCA (World Organization of National Colleges, Academies and Academic Associations of General
Practitioners/Family Physicians; shortened to World Organization of Family Doctors) was set up in 1972 as
a not-for-profit organization to represent family doctors and general practitioners around the world. It now
(2016) has a membership of around 500,000 family doctors from 131 countries; www.globalfamilydoctor.
com/AboutWonca/brief.aspx (accessed 14 June 2016).

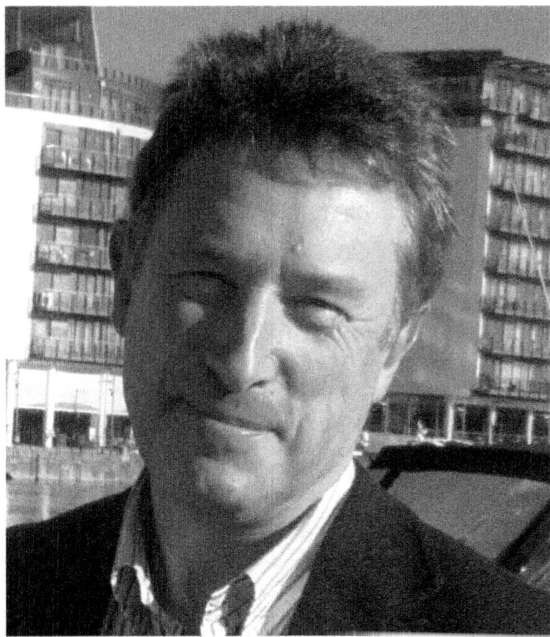

Figure 4: Dr John Wynn-Jones

the Working Party on Rural Practice of WONCA.[8] I was the first chair of the WONCA Working Party on Rural Practice, and was the chair until 2004. I'm pleased that we have all of the chairs of the Working Party on Rural Practice over the years with us today. So Jim Rourke, in Canada, took over from me, then Ian Couper in South Africa, and now John Wynn-Jones in Wales. So I'm going to open it up to go around the table and ask other people to make introductions. This Witness Seminar certainly is happening with the support and involvement of the WONCA Working Party on Rural Practice so maybe I'll ask John Wynn-Jones, the current chair of the working party, to start the ball rolling. So John, could you introduce yourself, please?

Dr John Wynn-Jones: I was a rural GP in mid-Wales. I started my time in general practice in mid-Wales in 1979, a long time ago. In those days we had no real access to any continuing professional development (CPD), and as a result of that I set up, with a colleague of mine, a local organization to run GP CPD in mid-Wales. This then expanded to setting up a rural doctors' group and we then set up the Rural GP Conference, which is held across the whole

---

[8] The Working Party on Rural Practice was set up in 1992; see the website at: www.globalfamilydoctor. com/groups/WorkingParties/RuralPractice.aspx (accessed 16 February 2016); for its history, see Couper *et al.* (2015). See also the discussion on page 147.

of the UK.[9] We're into our 25th-plus year of that, which will be held at the end of this month. I became interested in rural practice and I was fortunate enough to go to the WONCA conference in Hong Kong in 1995 and that really changed everything for me. I met all these activists around the world, I joined the WONCA Working Party, which was established formally in 1995, although the original group had got together in 1992. I went on to China to the first WONCA Rural World Conference in Shanghai in 1996[10] and I came back from that and felt that I needed to do something in Europe, and became involved with the Royal College of GPs where we had a small rural working group. But I took a chance in 1997 and gathered people that I knew across Europe and we established the first, and, until recently, the only regional rural doctors group called EURIPA (European Rural and Isolated Practitioners Association), and I was chair of that for 15 years.[11] I gave up the role in 2013 and rather probably foolishly took on the role of chairing the WONCA Working Party. Then we established a work stream for 2013 onwards for three years and we'll be coming to the end of that now, and I'm actually at the moment writing the report for WONCA executive for 2015. In addition to that I'm a senior lecturer in rural and global health at Keele University, and I'm still a part-time GP just working one day a week. It's been a great journey. I've been fortunate to travel around the world and I say to my medical students that, in fact, you can still be a rural GP in the middle of Wales and also work in an international capacity. So there's still life in the old dog and it has been a great experience.

Roger Strasser: Thank you very much, John, and welcome. Maybe if we keep with the theme of chairs of the Working Party and I see Ian Couper on screen, if you could introduce yourself now, Ian?

Professor Ian Couper: I'm Ian Couper from South Africa. I've been a rural doctor in a remote hospital, in Northern KwaZulu-Natal on the border of Mozambique, called Manguzi, for nine years.

---

[9] The Annual Rural Primary Care Conference (originally the Rural Doctors Conference) was set up by a group of GPs (the Montgomeryshire Medical Society) to address the educational needs of rural GPs. It was first held in 1990.

[10] See Strasser (1997).

[11] Established in 1997, EURIPA 'is a representative network organisation founded by family doctors to address the health and wellbeing needs of rural communities and the professional needs of those serving them across Europe. It represents a growing network of rural practitioners and organisations across Europe working together to disseminate good practice, initiate research and influence policy.' http://euripa. woncaeurope.org/ (accessed 16 March 2016).

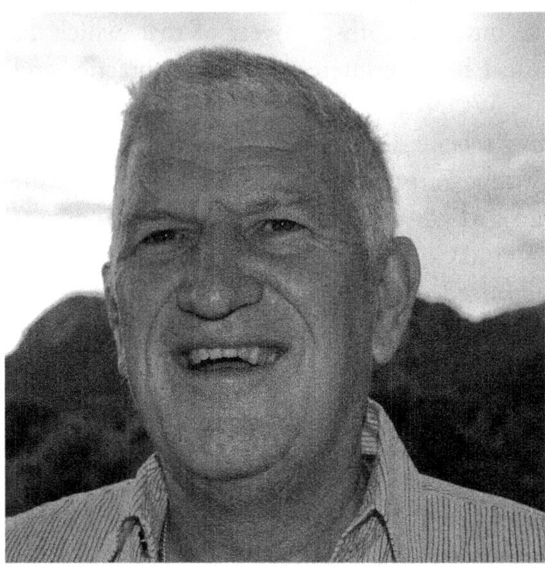

Figure 5: Professor Ian Couper

Since then I've been a rural doctor/family physician working in the North West Province, which is an inland province in South Africa, working in different capacities there. I was fortunate to attend the first International Conference on Rural Medicine in Shanghai in 1996 and have managed, in various ways and guises, to attend every single one of the rural health conferences since, which puts me in a small group with Roger and I'm not sure who else. But, yes, we've reached 13 conferences. In 1997, in South Africa, I was part of a group of doctors who formed the Rural Doctors Association of Southern Africa (RuDASA),[12] which was really formed in KwaZulu-Natal, which had quite a strong legacy of rural doctors coming out of rural mission hospitals in that area. The rural mission hospitals is a theme I'm sure we'll come back to because it's a major theme of rural medicine in South Africa. But it went across the country since then and is still going strong and in three weeks' time we will have our annual conference that's been happening every year since then. In 1998 I was fortunate to spend six months at the Monash Centre for Rural Health in Moe with Roger, and really that helped to develop some of my thinking. In 2000 I took a position at what was then called the Medical University of Southern Africa. It's gone through some name changes since then but that was where I had done

---

[12] The aim of the Rural Doctors Association of Southern Africa is 'for all rural people in Southern Africa to have access to quality health care'; The organization 'strives for the adequate staffing of rural health services by appropriately skilled medical staff and to be a voice for the rural doctor regarding training and working conditions.' www.rudasa.org.za/index.php/about/overview (accessed 16 March 2016).

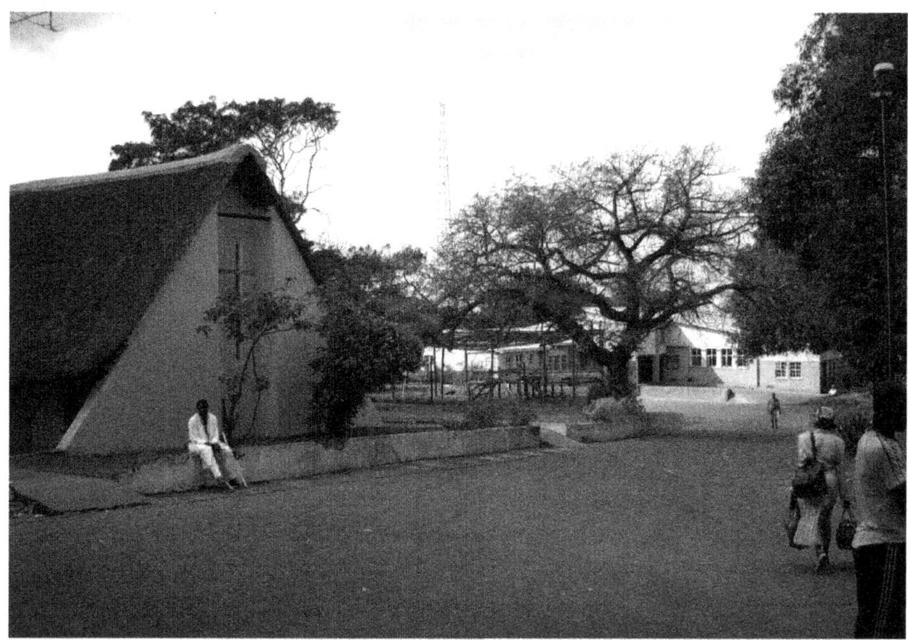

Figure 6: Manguzi Hospital

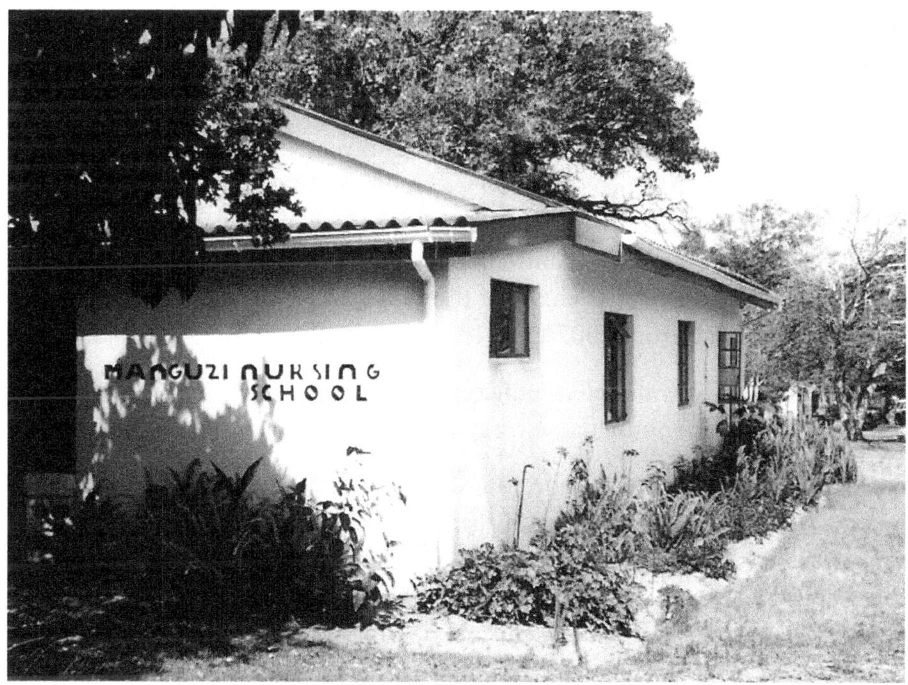

Figure 7: Manguzi Nursing School

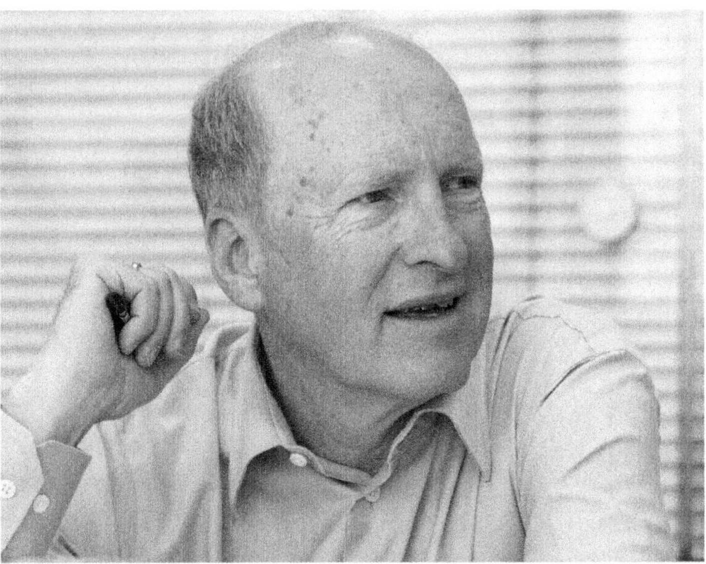

Figure 8: Professor James Rourke

my postgraduate family medicine studies in a decentralized training programme and that's what attracted me to go and work there – the decentralized nature of their training. In 2002, I was recruited by the University of the Witwatersrand, Wits University, to a position of Professor of Rural Health and became the first chair of rural health on the African continent in that position. I've been there until now as a joint appointment between the university and the provincial health service driving rural medicine and family medicine and primary care development in the province. In 2009 we established a Centre for Rural Health at Wits, which is continuing to develop and, in fact, next week we are having our annual rural health week and annual rural health seminar in the faculty. I'm also in the succession of chairs of the WONCA Working Party and Rural Practice; I was chair from 2007 to 2013.

Roger Strasser: To complete the picture of Working Party chairs, I'll ask Jim Rourke to introduce himself.

Professor James Rourke: I hope you can hear me all out across the world. It's so nice to be talking with all of you again. And thank you, Roger and Tilli, for setting this up. It's a pleasure to be here. I guess my rural experience goes back to being delivered by a rural doctor quite a few years ago, and I grew up on a farm in a very rural part of Canada, went to a one-room school house with all eight grades, one teacher with 25 students. I was the only student in my class for six years. So for me rural was normal until I went to university.

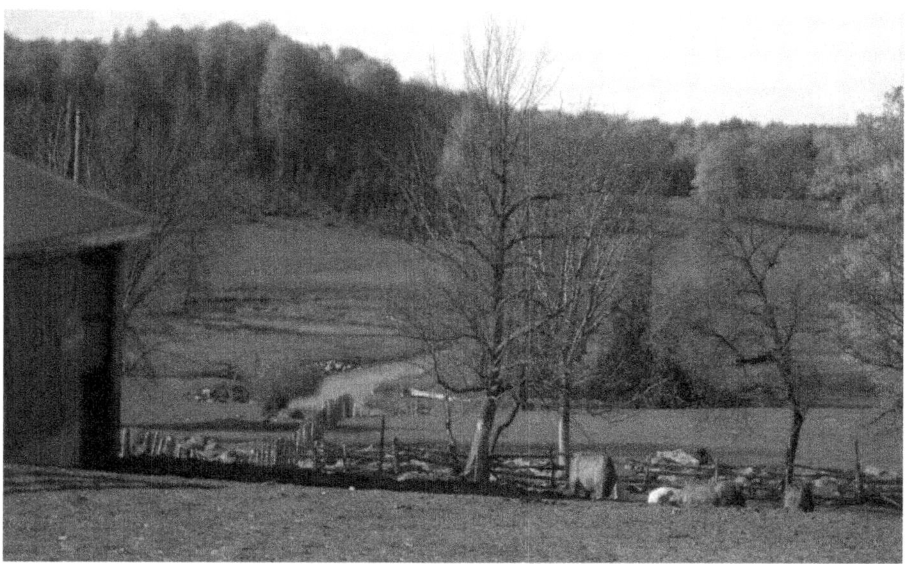

Figure 9: The Rourke family farm

When I went to university I realized the world was a bigger place, there were many different viewpoints on what rural was. I went into medical school and really had an eye on coming back to rural practice so did a lot of training at that time, picking and choosing what would work for that. I also met my wife, Leslie Rourke, who is also a rural family doctor, and although she had an urban background, her grandfather had practised rural medicine for 50 years in a small, rural town in Canada. So we had a rural background, a family background of rural medicine. We both set out in a career of rural medicine and when we graduated we spent 25 years in rural practice in a small community with very little specialist backup; we practised the whole textbook of rural medicine.

What became clear over time, and I'm sure we'll talk a bit more about it, was over the years the face of medicine changed, and I could see from a number of other people in Canada that the kind of training that was happening for family doctors was primarily urban-centred and they were no longer developing the skills needed for rural practice. So that prompted a number of us to start pushing for reform, and one of the things that came together was the 1992 Vancouver WONCA meeting, where I met Roger Strasser and a bunch of other keen people. I ended up taking an unpaid 'sabbatical' from rural practice, to join Roger and Sarah in Australia for six months in 1994, as Roger set up the Centre for Rural Health there. Then we came back to our rural practice and continued to pursue the idea at the University of Western Ontario, establishing a fairly

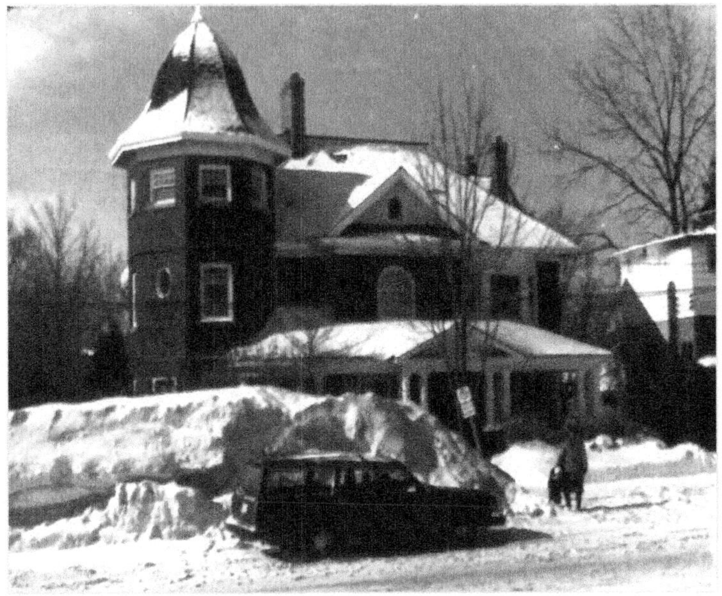

Figure 10: Leslie Rourke in front of Drs James and Leslie Rourke's
medical office in Goderich (Ontario)

broad rural medicine unit at the university, building on some of the principles that were being developed across the world at that time, with the same sort of ideas. We'll talk about that later. At the end of 25 years' rural practice and developing academic rural practice, I moved then to Memorial University in Newfoundland, to become the Dean of Medicine there. Memorial University of Newfoundland is in Canada's most rural province – 500,000 people spread over 400,000 km², or about the geographic size of the UK and Ireland and part of France put together but with a very small, widely distributed population. I've been involved there in rural practice and that's been quite a joy. I have managed to continue doing some rural practice in that time, some clinics in some sites and humanitarian work in Haiti to keep my hand in active rural practice because I find that does give some more credibility as well.

It's a joy to keep doing some rural practice as well as the medical school administration. All this time I've been involved with the Society of Rural Physicians of Canada from its beginning, which has been our Rural Doctors Association and trying to work with the College of Family Physicians of Canada, which is a group that looks after family medicine training standards in Canada, and trying to move everything towards better rural medical education across

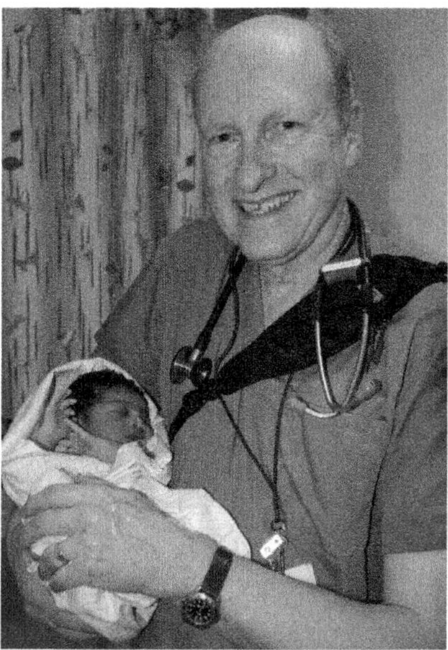

Figure 11: Professor James Rourke in Haiti

Canada.[13] I think we'll talk more as we go on about those different factors but that's a snapshot of my rural practice and life. My daughter's currently doing rural practice in British Columbia right now in a small town as a locum, so it's carrying on through the family, one could say, from Leslie's grandfather down to her, to me and our daughter.

Roger Strasser: We've now done all the chairs of the WONCA Working Party on Rural Practice, where do we go now? I'll ask Jo Scott-Jones to introduce himself next.

Dr Jo Scott-Jones: Thank you very much, Roger, and thank you for welcoming me as part of this group. I'm thrilled. So, like most New Zealand rural GPs, I'm from overseas. I trained in the UK then went to Australia to do a diploma in obstetrics, having qualified in 1986, because I thought that obstetrics was going to be an important part of family medicine and that was an opportunity to travel. I worked out a work visa in Australia and then came to New Zealand

---

[13] The Society of Rural Physicians of Canada is a voluntary professional organization founded in 1992. Its mission is 'to provide leadership for rural physicians and to promote sustainable conditions and equitable health care for rural communities'; www.srpc.ca/srpc_about.html (accessed 5 September 2016). The College of Family Physicians of Canada, founded in 1954, is a national medical association and the professional organization responsible 'for establishing standards for the training, certification and lifelong education of family physicians and for advocating on behalf of the specialty of family medicine, family physicians and their patients'; www.cfpc.ca/AboutUs/ (accessed 5 September 2016).

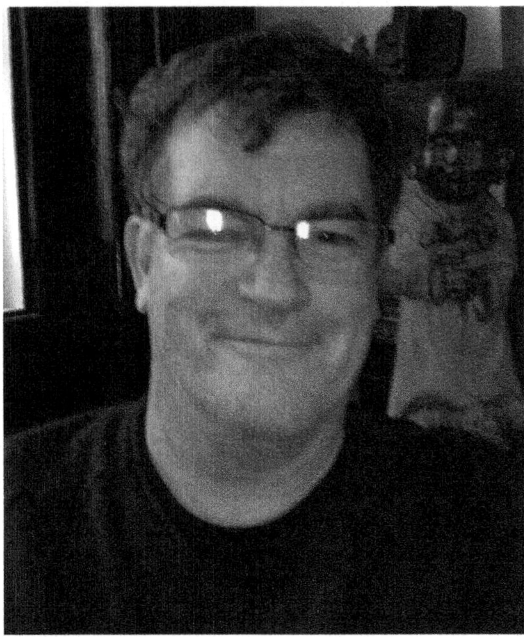

Figure 12: Dr Jo Scott-Jones

for six months – that was 23 years ago. I landed in Opotiki, which is a small, rural town on the east coast, and found work that was immensely satisfying with the breadth of practice that we all know is characteristic of rural work in a very high-needs community. Having been brought up in the centre of Liverpool in the UK, I'd always seen myself as being an inner city GP. But, on reflection, I think that was because of the desire to serve a high-needs community and I certainly have that in the work that I do. In terms of my involvement with rural education and the development of colleges, working backwards, I've been the inaugural chair of our New Zealand Rural Health Alliance, which started two years ago, bringing together 35 organizations who are interested in rural health and well-being across New Zealand, from professional and community and industry organizations.[14] I'm the immediate past chair of the New Zealand Rural General Practice Network, which was set up in the early 1990s – an offshoot of the New Zealand Medical Association – again developed really as a response to rural GPs recognizing a difference in culture and a difference in need

---

[14] RHAANZ (Rural Health Alliance Aotearoa New Zealand) was established in 2012, the main objective to 'bring a "united voice" – from across multiple rural sector organisations – to develop solutions and influence policy affecting the health and wellbeing of rural communities'; www.rhaanz.org.nz/about-us/our-objectives/ (accessed 16 March 2016).

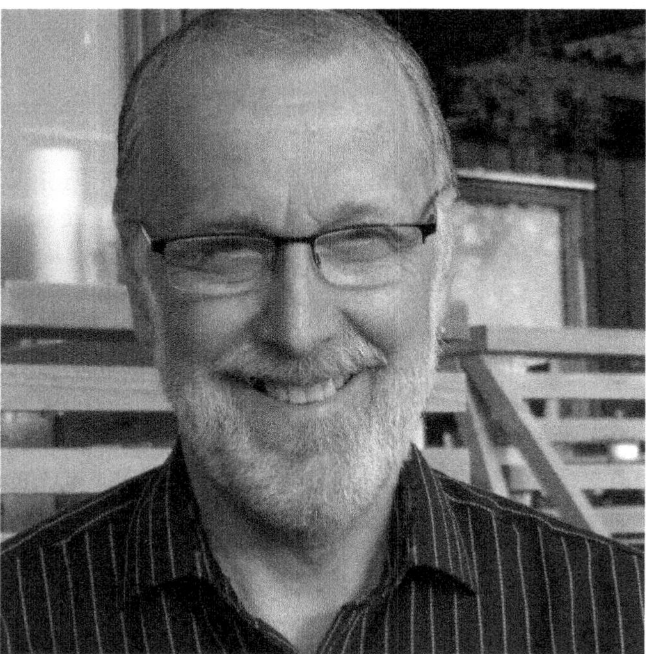

Figure 13: Professor Ivar Aaraas

from the urban colleagues, at that time, around a particular political issue.[15] The New Zealand Rural Practice Network has been a supportive organization that has driven the agenda in rural health for New Zealand since that time. I'm also currently the chair of the Rural Faculty of the College of GPs of New Zealand, which was only established in the 1970s, which I think is when this history seminar is aimed to begin. The Rural Faculty has a Division of the Fellowship of Rural Hospital Medicine as well, which is again quite a new organization that represents another change in the way that we train our rural providers in New Zealand.

Roger Strasser: Thanks for the reminder – as we get into the conversation the focus is on the period from 1970 to 2000, in terms of the history of medicine.

Professor Ivar Aaraas: Thank you for inviting me. I'm talking from Tromsø, in the far north of Norway, where I started my career in 1970. After graduation at the University of Oslo, I moved to the north to serve my obligatory internship. In 1970 a new university, including a medical school, was about to be started in Tromsø. My medical and rural history is much connected to the history of the

---

[15] See their website at www.rgpn.org.nz/Home.aspx (accessed 16 March 2016).

medical school of Tromsø from 1970 to 2000.[16] At an early stage, the founding Dean, Peter F Hjort, travelled around the world and studied various innovative models of medical education, which had recently been introduced in Canada (McMaster), Israel (Be'er Sheva), and the Netherlands (Maastricht).[17] He adopted many elements from those models into the new curriculum in Tromsø, which was much oriented towards developing healthcare for people in the northern region of Norway. Up to 1970, Northern Norway was in many ways left behind as an underprivileged, rural region of the country, particularly with respect to standards of education and health. The mission of Peter Hjort was to do something about this, to create equity and justice for people in Northern Norway. To come here in 1970 and be part of the development of that medical school from the beginning was a fantastic start to my career. During my internship period I was lucky to meet my future wife Ann-Mari. She was in the second class of Tromsø medical students starting in 1974. I followed her studies from 1974 to 1980 while I was working as a GP in the city of Tromsø. Actually, Tromsø with the university campus is the most urban part of Northern Norway. After Ann-Mari graduated, we left Tromsø and settled in a northern rural community, where we worked together as GPs for 12 years, before we returned to Tromsø to start different further careers. She specialized as a psychiatrist, while I started an academic career with the main emphasis on medical education and research in rural areas. At the University I was appointed a lecturer and coordinator for the placement of the medical students in rural communities. Since the beginning, Tromsø students have spent most of the fifth year (of a total of six years) away from the campus in rural areas, in local hospitals and in primary care with GPs. Before I started as a coordinator I'd had experience as a teacher/mentor for students in my own rural practice for many years. During the following years, along with organizing and coordinating student placements all over Northern Norway, I finished my PhD thesis, a study about use and usefulness of small rural community hospitals. Through this educational and scientific activity I was later engaged to lead the planning of a new National Centre of Rural Medicine, affiliated with the University of Tromsø. When the Centre was officially established in 2007, I was appointed as its first head and professor. After I retired in 2013, I have continued in a part-time engagement with the Centre as professor emeritus/senior adviser.

---

[16] Aaraas and Halvorsen (2014).

[17] Professor Peter Hjort (1924–2011) was a Norwegian physician with interests in haematology, public health, geriatrics, and gerontology. He was instrumental in establishing the University of Tromsø, of which he was the first Rector from 1972 to 1973; https://en.wikipedia.org/wiki/Peter_F._Hjort (accessed 8 June 2016).

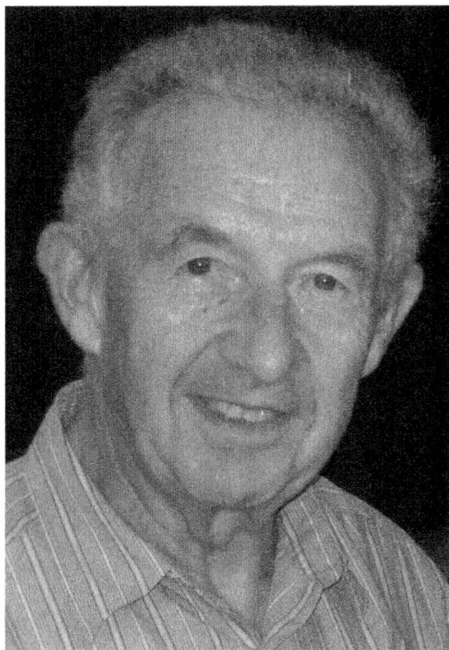

Figure 14: Professor John Hamilton

Roger Strasser: I've already mentioned John Hamilton, who is in Australia today, or tonight.

Professor John Hamilton: I'm the odd ball amongst you. I'm actually a specialist physician when I'm in my natural circumstance. I qualified in 1960 in England and after two years went for my first dose of rural medicine, with two years completely immersed in rural Zambia in a mission hospital. Notwithstanding my training as a physician, I found myself doing hysterectomies, craniotomies, paediatrics, the whole boiling lot – and was sometimes the only doctor within 100 km in any direction. One of the big lessons I learned was that you needed to get into the villages, listen, and see their point of view. That stayed with me because it had a lot of impact in some of the later medical schools I was involved with. I returned in culture shock back to Hammersmith Hospital and then moved on to research in small bowel physiology at Barts, and then got scooped up to go to McMaster University at its beginning, and I was one of the junior members of the faculty there. I found myself chairing the student selection committee and then the curriculum committee and that's where problem-based learning was put together.[18] The history on the ground is not exactly as it was

---

[18] See, for example, Spaulding (1969).

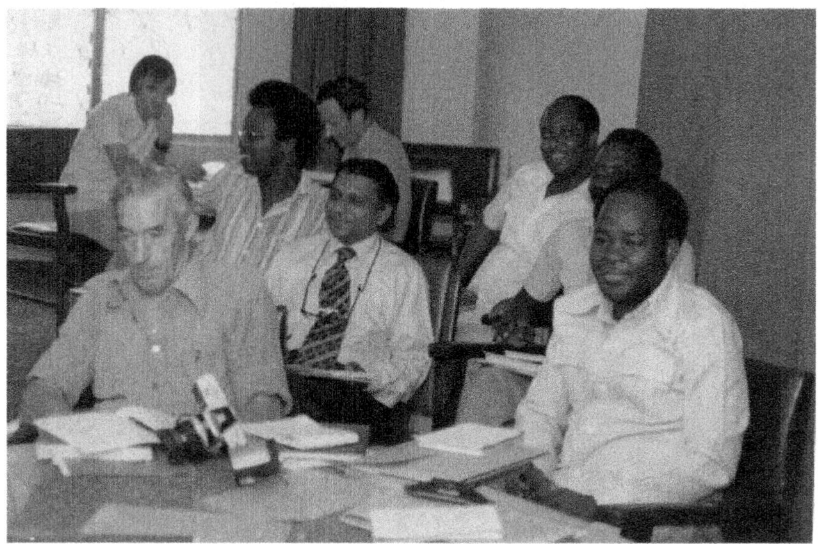

Figure 15: Ilorin WHO workshop to launch the Curriculum (1978)

described. It's described by others, looking in retrospect at it, but that's not what we're here for tonight. That's where population medicine, clinical epidemiology, and the David Sackett evidence-based medicine was shaping itself.[19] After that, married with children, we decided we'd go and take ourselves to Nigeria, and I was Professor of Medicine, but more particularly, chair of the curriculum of the Ilorin Medical School, set up in the wake of a new policy change to have primary healthcare extended throughout rural regions.

We placed our students in villages to live there day and night for a month every year. The same village, different seasons, so they had a five-year bonding experience with a specific community that had never been studied before, and they learned a great deal by their studies of health and disease causes, what we would call now the social determinants of health. We didn't know those words and we couldn't buy airline tickets to go to posh conferences. In fact we couldn't even make a phone call. I've met those graduates 20–30 years later – some of them at the Calabar WONCA rural conference – and that experience has stayed with them all the way through. It gave them a much wider perspective on where their medical role was.

---

[19] Dr David Sackett (1934–2015) was a leading proponent of evidence-based medicine. He defined it as 'the conscientious, explicit, and judicious use of current best evidence in making decisions about the care of individual patients. The practice of evidence-based medicine means integrating individual clinical expertise with the best available external clinical evidence from systematic research': Sackett *et al.* (1996). For David Sackett, see Smith (2015).

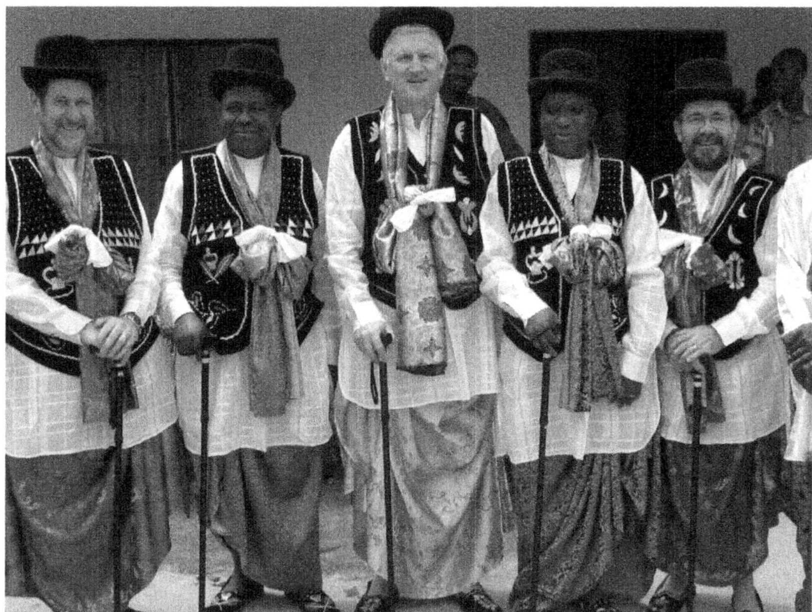

Figure 16: WONCA Rural Conference in Calabar; those awarded an honorary chieftainship in the Okoyong Council of Traditional Rulers and Chiefs, Cross River State, Nigeria in February 2008 (from left to right: Roger Strasser, Ndifreke Udonwa, Ian Couper, Victor Inem, Bruce Chater

From there, I went to the World Bank for a period in the Population, Health and Nutrition Division and then was asked to go to Australia, to Newcastle. That was the medical school set up specifically with a government mandate to try new things, to get out into social aspects of medicine and medical education, and that we were doing – we were well into rural areas before most of the other schools had really made those moves. Soon after starting there, to my surprise, I was asked to be the founding chair of the new Australian Medical Council (AMC) Accreditation Committee, and I took great care to make sure that we always had a representative of community medicine or general practice on every accrediting body, because that was the area that others could not speak for. So that worked well. I know, because the president of the AMC wrote later about it, that the reason I was asked to do it newly arrived was they did not want somebody from the establishment.[20] They wanted somebody who had different views. A bit of a risk for a new Dean of a wacky medical school to be given that sort of position, but it worked.

---

[20] Professor John Hamilton wrote: 'The President stated that this is a limited circulation account.' Email to Ms Caroline Overy, 8 November 2016.

Soon after I started, I was asked to chair the Rural Undergraduate Steering Committee (RUSC), which was part of a larger initiative to improve rural healthcare, and this section of it was through undergraduate medical education. That's where Roger and I, and many other good people, first met. I've just re-read the report – that's the RUSC report in 1994 – and we put in, in fact I wrote these words myself, that it was not just enough for students to learn to give healthcare in a rural setting, but they had to get into the rural community and become part of it, like they did in Nigeria.[21] There was precedent in Australia with the Hawkesbury Agricultural College, where their curriculum was as much the community of the agricultural world as it was agricultural science.[22] I was also chair of the Commonwealth Study of Women Embedded in Practice, particularly focused on rural, which explored many, many issues that were preventing women going into or feeling comfortable in rural practice. It was a complex issue. I was also chairing the Diarrheal Diseases Control Program for the World Health Organization, and that led us to change the way we looked at the implementation of a scientifically based programme in communities when we found that it was actually stopping people using the natural remedies they had, which were actually better for early oral rehydration, not because they were chemically right but because they were socially available and immediately available.[23]

And so it went on. I then went to Durham in the north of England, and that's where we put the students outside the health service and into the welfare sector as the way of getting them into the real world. We were in an urban setting, post-industrial collapse of coal mining, steelworks, and so on. But really the approach is the same if you go, for example, into the centre of Wales during the awful time when all the farming collapsed and so on. The social agendas that need to be addressed are beyond the range that usually we think of as health. So you need these partnerships in the welfare sector. And I'm doing that now. I still chair the last two years of our curriculum and I'm putting students for a month's immersion into welfare sector programmes, and they're using the same language as the students in Nigeria; that is, they had never seen that world for what it is. They could not have imagined it. Now they have a sympathetic point of

---

[21] Commonwealth Department of Human Services and Health (1994).

[22] Hawkesbury Agricultural College, the first agricultural college in New South Wales, was established in 1892.

[23] Professor John Hamilton was a Member and Chairman of the Technical Advisory Group of the WHO Diarrheal Diseases Control Program from 1987 to 1991.

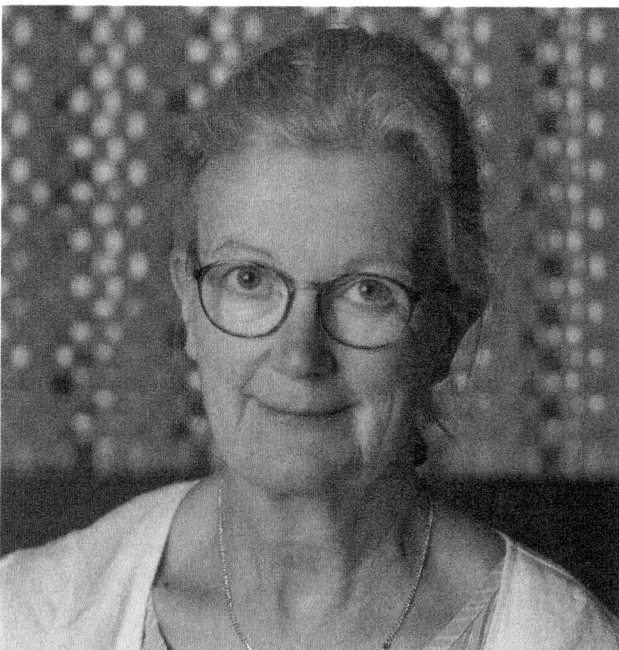

Figure 17: Professor Sarah Strasser

view, they understand the situation of homeless people, drug addicts, prisoners coming out, and so on. I do feel that, be it urban or be it rural, you've got to get beyond the medical boundary to see what the real world is. You've got to work through other people's eyes, the welfare sector, that sort of thing. I've seen back in Durham, where it was very difficult to get any general practitioners, if you go into this difficult industrial area, several of those graduates, 15 years down the line, have now formed networks in practice in those settings. They meet monthly and it's because they've got into the community they felt bonded to it, they could see the other support groups that you would hardly see if you stayed in the medical circle. They knew how to work with them. End of sermon. [Laughter] I'm the oldest, I'm the least suitable for rural practice of all of you.

Roger Strasser: Well, your description of your time in Zambia hardly agrees with your self-description, I have to say. You mentioned women in rural practice, so maybe we'll ask Sarah Strasser to introduce herself at this time.

Professor Sarah Strasser: Hello everyone. In 1970 I was still at high school but quite determined to be a rural GP at that point because both my parents and my grandfather were rural GPs and I knew that was where I wanted to go. By the 2000s we were in Australia and had five children and I'd worked in rural UK, rural Canada, and rural Australia. So it's been quite a journey, even for those relatively few years. I was thinking, listening to everyone else, how interesting it all is, and thank you for organizing this conference call. We went through a number of eye-opening things that I just thought I'd emphasize, although they have been mentioned by other people. For us as rural practitioners, not having any support or understanding of what was going on out there, it made a huge difference to go to the early start of continuing education programmes, specifically designed for rural physicians and incorporating support for partners, and the rural GPs' families. So I became part of the rural network in Australia for women and families supporting partners. I was also obviously part of the group as a rare female rural GP and also part of the overseas-trained group. So I've touched on a lot of the things that you have all spoken about. I guess the biggest impact that I feel I've had with regard to rural practice is really around rural education. I've been associated with starting new rural education programmes over the years, trying to basically bring in common sense where things seem to have got out of hand. I brought my Canadian experience of being a trainee in a practice over a long period of time, so that in Australia we were able to set up an opportunity for GP registrars to stay in one practice for their whole postgraduate training and develop some of the links that I think your students were finding, John [Hamilton], by living and working in the community for a long period of time. I was also involved in establishing the then Pilot Remote Vocational Training Stream, which was about making sure a community would not lose their rural doctor because they had to go off and train somewhere else, moving around every few months.[24] We set up this remote training programme to give them support to stay where they were and serve their communities. I think the other thing I was just going to say was that, after all these years in the business, I've picked up more and more of the social accountability and advocacy role, so that I have been more and more involved in working in education with regard to training others to better care for Aboriginal people, and have had wonderful opportunities myself to get to know Aboriginal communities better. So really I just want to say, thank you very much for rekindling all these memories as much as anything.

---

[24] Founded in 1999, the Pilot Remote Vocational Training Stream (PRVTS) was 'a joint initiative of the Royal Australian College of General Practitioners (RACGP) and the Australian College of Rural and Remote Medicine (ACRRM) … to provide vocational training to general practitioners in remote areas, who would otherwise have difficulty accessing training'; www.rvts.org.au/about/history (accessed 16 March 2016). Following its success, it was renamed the Remote Vocational Training Scheme in 2003. For the career paths of the Remote Vocational Training Scheme registrars see Wearne *et al.* (2010).

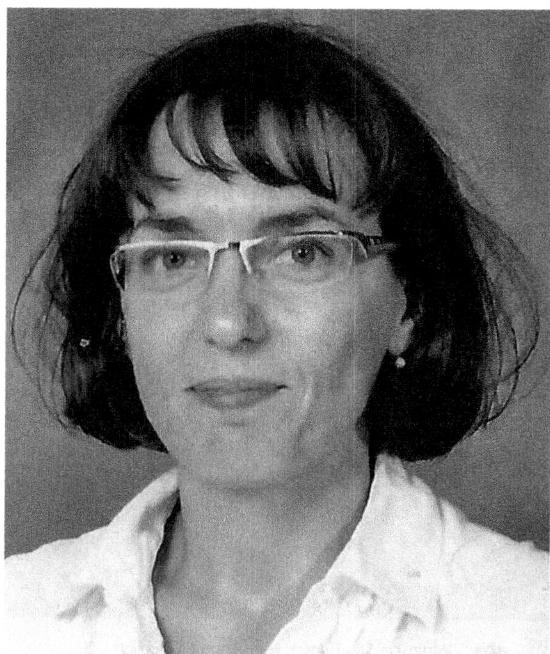

Figure 18: Professor Maja Račić

Roger Strasser: Let's go back around the world, maybe Maja Račić, you would introduce yourself?

Professor Maja Račić: So hello to everyone, thank you for inviting me to attend this Seminar. I'm working as a Vice-Dean for a small medical school, which is actually in a rural area of Bosnia Herzegovina. I used to work as a rural GP but I could say that I'm working as a rural professor right now. The mission of my school is to develop rural medicine because around 60 per cent of the area in Bosnia Herzegovina is rural. It's very important to change the quality of the services that we're offering to our patients. Many of my residents come from a rural region and through the training, which is partly urban and partly in a rural region, we are trying to change the concept of family medicine because, even though we have been going through reform of primary healthcare for the last 15 years, we still have a lot of problems. For centuries, not just for the last few decades, doctors in Bosnia Herzegovina, health insurance companies, and the Ministry of Health have focused more on secondary than primary healthcare. So it's really very expensive and it's not a suitable model for the country, which is still developing. So through development of rural family medicine we are trying also to develop family medicine within the country. Also I just recently joined

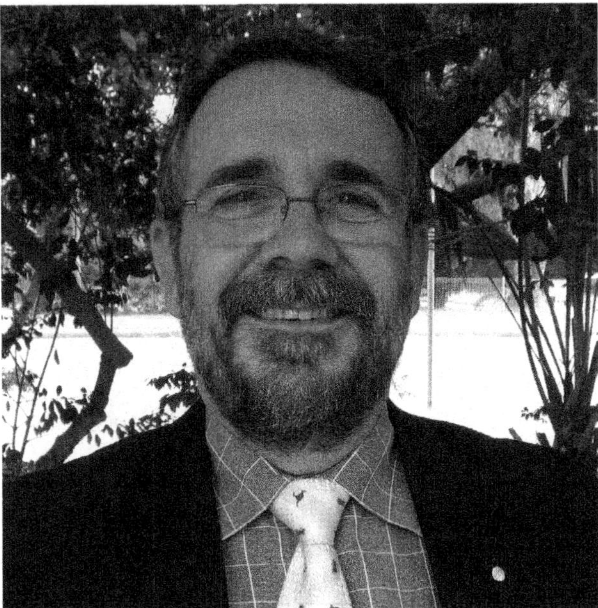

Figure 19. Professor Bruce Chater

the rural WONCA party. I do not have such interesting stories as you have – I haven't been working in Zambia or in interesting parts of the world – but we are trying to do the best we can here.

Roger Strasser: Where you are is a very interesting part of the world and we're very pleased to have you with us today.

Professor Bruce Chater: It's a great pleasure to be with so many friends tonight, our time, and afternoon your time. I first moved to the little town of Theodore, which is 600 km from our capital and the nearest very large specialist centre, in 1981, and was involved since then doing obstetrics and anaesthetics. We had a bit of a clash with our Government in the 1980s about our terms and conditions because they basically expected us to work for very little to keep a hospital open in rural areas. Also, we were very interested in education and training for rural practice, which really didn't exist at that time except through people making *ad hoc* training plans. In 1989 we formed the Rural Doctors Association and I was the initial secretary of that in our state of Queensland.[25] I'm very proud to say that my wife also at that stage formed a rural family group to support the families of rural practitioners and that was part of the charter of

---

[25] See the website of the Rural Doctors Association of Queensland at www.rdaq.com.au/en-au/home.aspx (accessed 21 March 2016).

the Rural Doctors Association. In 1991 we held, at the request of the National Minister for Health, the first National Rural Health Conference, which set up the first Australian policy framework in rural health, and from that conference we formed, and I was the founding convenor of, the Rural Doctors Association of Australia.[26] I was then the first chair of the National Rural Health Alliance, which brings together all the bodies with an interest in rural health, from nurses through to pharmacists and others.[27] At the conference we, as rural doctors, talked to the College of General Practitioners as I was in fact on their council in 1994 to set up a rural faculty. After some ructions and difficulties, in 1997 the Australian College of Rural and Remote Medicine (ACRRM) was formed, and we now have two general practice colleges in Australia, with the ACRRM obviously having a rural emphasis.[28] I was the president of the ACRRM from 2003 to 2005 and moved on with them from there. With respect to WONCA, I joined the WONCA working party at a very exciting time in Hong Kong in 1995 and was privileged to go to Beijing with Roger Strasser to talk to the Chinese Association about running the 1996 Shanghai conference, the first international conference on rural and remote health.[29] From those conferences we developed the WONCA policy on rural and remote health, which actually coalesced all the recommendations from several conferences in a summary and was complementary to the document that I don't think has been mentioned so far but was the first document on training for rural practice, which the initial group started in 1992.[30] Just over recent times I've been appointed an Associate Professor of Rural and Remote Medicine at the University of Queensland in 2005, and helped start the rural generalist programme, which is now training 80 rural doctors with extended skills and general practice skills for rural and remote practice in our state of Queensland in Australia.

---

[26] The first National Rural Health Conference 'A Fair go for Rural Health' was held in February 1991 at Toowoomba, Queensland. The proceedings are available online at: http://ruralhealth.org.au/1stNRHC/1_ CONPRO.PDF (accessed 21 March 2016). The Rural Doctors Association of Australia (RDAA) is '… a national body representing the interests of rural medical practitioners right around Australia. [Their] vision is for excellent medical care for rural and remote communities'; www.rdaa.com.au/about-us (accessed 21 March 2016). See also comments on page 146.

[27] See the website of the National Rural Health Alliance at http://www.ruralhealth.org.au/about (accessed 21 March 2016). For the history and development of the organization, see Chater (1993).

[28] See, for example, Nichols, Streeton, and Cowie (2002).

[29] See note 10.

[30] WONCA Working Party on Rural Practice (1995).

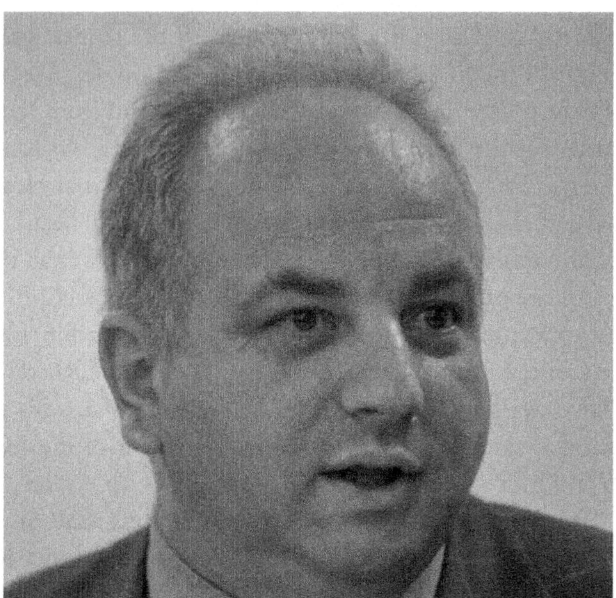

Figure 20: Professor Petar Bulat

Professor Petar Bulat: Thank you for inviting me to the conference. I am an occupational health doctor, mostly dealing with occupational health issues. My interest in rural health arose when I met Professor Miodrag Milošević, one of the founders of rural health in the region of Serbia and former Yugoslavia.[31] Through contact with him I got interested in rural health, mainly in the field of occupational toxicology as I'm dealing with people exposed to pesticides, so this was my primary interest in the rural health topic. Then in 2002 I met Claudio Colosio at a conference that he organized in Bari (Italy) and after it, with his help, I organized a conference here in Belgrade on rural health issues with a focus on the south-east of Europe.[32] After it, with the support of Claudio Colosio at the International Commission on Occupational Health (ICOH) Conference in Milan (Italy) in 2006, I became the Secretary of the Rural Health Scientific Committee of ICOH until 2012. At the moment we are preparing for the next conference in Lodi (Italy), which we will have next

---

[31] Professor Petar Bulat added: 'I mentioned Professor Miodrag Milošević due to his very important role in rural health development in Serbia. He was Professor of Hygiene at University of Belgrade School of Medicine but he also had an Occupational Health Specialist degree. He was very active in international societies dealing with rural health and one of the leaders in the Balkan region. He died in 2007.' Email to Ms Caroline Overy, 8 June 2016.

[32] Claudio Colosio is Associate Professor of Occupational Health in the Department of Occupational and Environmental Health at the University of Milan.

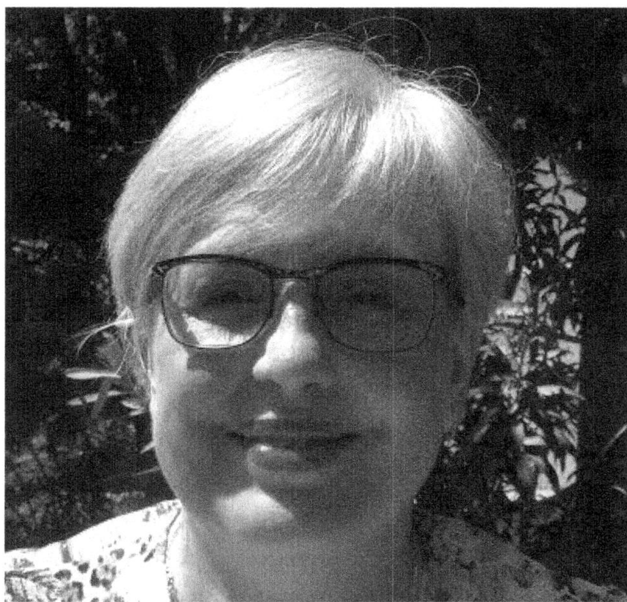

Figure 21: Dr Tanja Pekez-Pavlisko

week. In the meantime the Serbian Academy of Sciences asked me to join their body, which is focused on developing rural areas; so for the last two years I have been working with them on developing rural areas, and we had a meeting last year at the Academy on rural health and I am privileged to have had as a guest here in Belgrade a colleague from Croatia, Tanja Pekez-Pavlisko. So I am more and more involved in rural health but I am not working as a rural health doctor myself. My context in rural health problems is mostly with people exposed to pesticides as I'm working at the National Institute for Occupational Health and running the Clinical Department of Occupational Toxicology.

Roger Strasser: Of course, a lot of rural health is occupational health because the occupations of people in rural areas are quite often risky and dangerous. You mention agriculture, mining, forestry, fishery, and so on, so that's certainly part of rural health. You mentioned Tanja, so maybe we'll ask Tanja to introduce herself.

Dr Tanja Pekez-Pavlisko: Thank you very much, Petar, for your introduction and thank you very much for inviting me to take part in this conference call; it is very important for all of us. Actually I come from part of Croatia, but was born in Bosnia Herzegovina. I hope that every one of you knows that one of the core establishers of the World Health Organization, Andrija Stampar, was born in Croatia. I finished my medical school in Banja Luka, which is in

Bosnia Herzegovina, where I was born, then I moved to Croatia and started my residency in emergency medicine – that was my first love. I left Zagreb because of the war,[33] and married here and had two children. For the first 15 years, during the war and after the war, I was working as an emergency physician in the prehospital department (ambulance). I introduced to Croatia, International Trauma Life Support courses in a role of Medical Director for Croatia for three years. I also participated in the organization of the first Mass Casualty course in Novalja, on the island of Pag. It started with a course in a rural setting, which was a medical response to a major incident, run by Sten Lennquist, a professor from Sweden, and Boris Hreckovski, from Croatia. After that I moved to family medicine and worked 70 km away from Zagreb. I'm now in solo practice 40 km away from the nearest hospital, which is a long distance in Croatia and in Europe. At this moment, I am Vice-Chair of the WONCA Working Party on Rural Practice, I organized the WONCA World Conference in Dubrovnik this year, and I'm president of the organizing committee of KoHOM (Croatian Family Physicians Coordination) conferences. KoHOM is the biggest organization of family physicians in Croatia, and I'm president of conferences of this organization, which has about 800 participants each year. What I like to do is palliative care, I have good connections with women's shelters so we are taking care of victims of domestic violence.

Roger Strasser: Let's come back to the room here, I'll ask Jim Douglas to introduce himself.

Dr James Douglas: I'm going to use my proper name, James Douglas, just to avoid any confusion with Jim Rourke who is sitting beside me. My career trajectory has been similar to several people who have already spoken. I've been a rural GP in a small town called Fort William, in the Highlands of Scotland, for the past 35 years. My career has really been to stay in one place and to continue to practise as a rural GP but also to pursue a role, which I see as really like a rural clinical scientist. I'm still currently full time, so I'm doing three days a week as a clinical GP – I was seeing patients all day yesterday. The other two days I do a mixture of management, education, and research. I don't have any university connections because the way that medicine is organized in the UK is slightly different from other parts of the world in that our postgraduate education is done by Royal Colleges and so on, rather than undergraduate universities. I currently have responsibilities for running the postgraduate GP rural fellowship scheme in Scotland, and also have responsibilities for general practice specialist training

---

[33] The Croatian War of Independence (1991–1995).

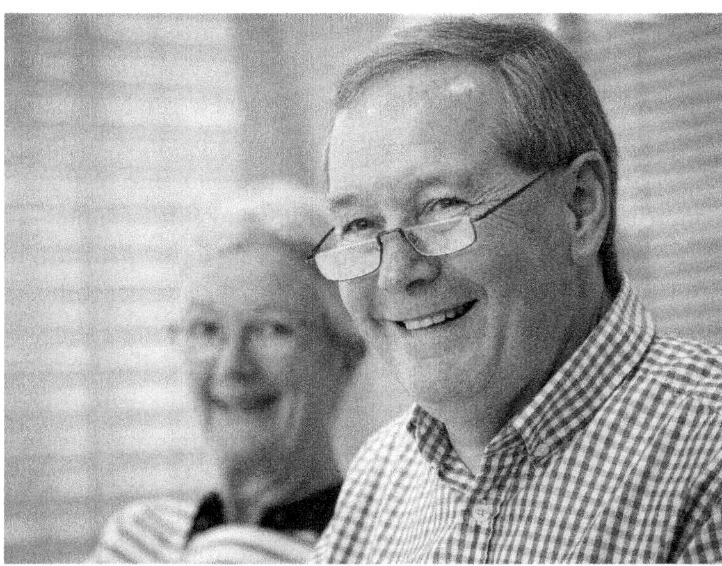

Figure 22: Professor Sarah Strasser and Dr James Douglas

within the UK and the current challenges of recruiting and retaining generation Y, which we can maybe come on to in the discussion later. In the time period from 1970 to 2000 that we're thinking of for the meeting here, if I reflect back on that, I went to Aberdeen University, which is one of the ancient universities of the UK. It was founded in 1495, so when I went there they'd already been training people to be doctors for 500 years. In 1970, at the start of this time period, I was an undergraduate in Aberdeen and rural experience was really regarded as normal and not very much different. So, in other words, the hinterland of the university city had lots of rural placements and it was regarded as quite normal and nothing different to be sent to a small community hospital, or be sent up to the Orkney Islands, or things like that. At that time, I didn't come from a rural background, and my track into rural practice was through sport. At that stage as an undergraduate I was a very keen scuba diver, and into water sports – sailing and diving. So my interest in becoming a rural GP started in Aberdeen at that time. There were very strong undergraduate role models of general practice and there was a well-established department of general practice in Aberdeen in 1970. So I came to the fairly naive, but fulfilled, conclusion that I wanted to be a GP on the west coast of Scotland where I could go diving. And that's really what I did. I took the active process of moving to Fort William, where I'm still a GP, in 1979. The attraction of that was there was a diving school, which had been established for training people for the North Sea at that stage, and I was the naive young boy, or young doctor, who already knew a little bit about diving. I went to a rural community to fulfil, if you like, a new rural need and I also had an academic interest, so I published quite a few papers on diving hyperbaric medicine.[34] That then took me, living in that rural community, to new rural industries. In the 1980s aquacultural fish farming was starting up so I became the first doctor, I think probably in the world, but I'm not 100 per cent sure of that, to define the occupational health problems of aquaculture and fish farming.[35] That took me into research into occupational asthma, observing in my patients in my own community, that several patients who'd started working at a new fish factory had developed asthma.[36] I then pursued that whole thing of being a clinical scientist and my current clinical interest in research is Lyme disease. If we're taking things right the way up to a little bit beyond 2000, I've seen a most definite increase and prevalence in Lyme borreliosis in my patients in my community – again, it's about living in a rural community and seeing things around you.[37] I'm now part of a new project called LymeMap, which is funded by the European Space Agency, and it's about trying to get a sort of risk prediction tool on to people's mobile phones.[38] Only last Tuesday I was involved in a community workshop, which was about how this research can be designed and what the app looks like, that sort of thing. So I suppose my career has been very much to sit within my rural community, to try to be as good as I can be, a doctor and general practitioner, also to educate young doctors and young nurses, but also to pursue this idea about the rural clinical scientist. And I've thoroughly enjoyed that career. One of the frustrations at the moment is that nobody now wants to do that career and, despite practising in a fantastic building, having all the facilities that I want, all the support that I need, we are currently in a situation where we're one down in my practice and we've been unable to recruit, to fulfil the position that I'm currently doing and have done for the past 12 months.[39] So we're in quite a challenge in general practice within the UK for a whole variety of reasons – we might be able to come back to that later.

---

[34] See, for example, Douglas (1985).

[35] Douglas and Milne (1991).

[36] Douglas *et al.* (1995). See Dr James Douglas' comments on asthma on page 111.

[37] For a summary of Lyme disease by James Douglas, 'Lyme borreliosis – a tricky diagnosis', see the Medical and Dental Defence Union of Scotland (MDDUS) website at www.mddus.com/resources/resource-type/ publications/summons/2016/spring-2016/lyme-borreliosis-a-tricky-diagnosis/ (accessed 1 June 2016).

[38] The European Space Agency gave €250,000 to LymeMap, a project to develop a mobile phone app to increase awareness and enable information, data, and location 'hotspots' of the disease to be uploaded; https://artes-apps.esa.int/projects/lymemap (accessed 23 March 2016).

[39] The problems of GP recruitment are also discussed by Dr Gordon Baird on pages 132–3.

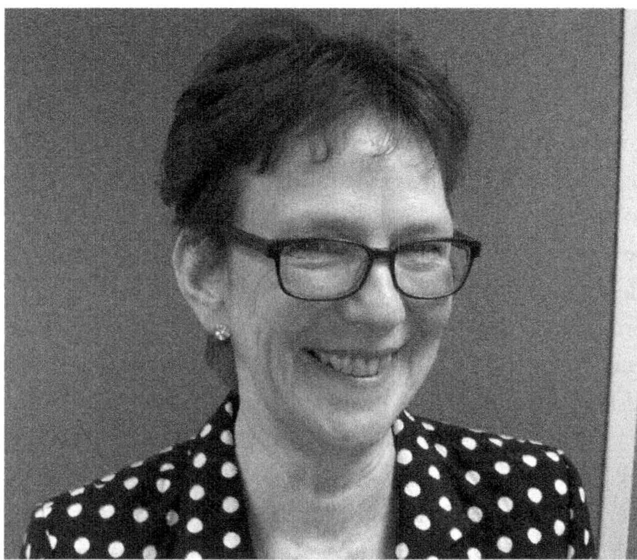

Figure 23: Ms Jane Randall-Smith

Despite having the best job, I think, in the world, nobody wants to follow in my footsteps. I've got four children: two of them are artists and two of them are medical. One is a specialist surgeon in ENT and one is a specialist psychiatrist in learning disability, so I haven't been terribly successful in inspiring my children in rural careers. With regard to the wider aspects, I've been very involved with the Royal College of General Practitioners in the United Kingdom and for a relatively short time I was involved in WONCA Rural Working Party and I was led into that by my good friend, John MacLeod, who was one of the original people who established the WONCA Rural Working Party with Roger Strasser and Jim Rourke and Bruce Chater and others.[40] I'm not currently a member of the WONCA Rural Working Party but I'm certainly still very active in the academic side here with the College and with training.

Ms Jane Randall-Smith: I feel very honoured to be here today because I'm actually a scientist by training and it was in 1996 that John Wynn-Jones asked if I would like to work with him to see if his idea for a centre for rural health was viable. Little did we know where that was going to go. I certainly didn't imagine I would be doing this today. But I worked with John at the Institute

---

[40] Dr John MacLeod (1935–2009) was a GP on the Hebridean Island of North Uist from 1973 until his retirement in 2000. As well as serving the island community, he sat on local, national, and international medical committees and was active in the Royal College of General Practitioners. See Douglas (2009). See also discussion of John MacLeod on pages 106–7.

[of Rural Health] from 1996 to 2012,[41] and although for a lot of it we really felt we were fighting an uphill struggle, we did have some significant achievements, and probably the greatest was rural proofing for health.[42] And although that's been picked up in other countries as well, we still have issues here and central Government is not really taking on rural issues, and I'm sure we'll pick that up later. We also worked very hard to get medical students and young doctors into rural practice and Richard [Hays] was involved with Keele on that. We still have medical students coming out and spending a significant amount of time in rural practice in Shropshire, which is just across the border from where I am now. In Wales it's been much more challenging, but I think it is beginning to happen. It shows you how long it takes to make changes take place. When we started the Institute, I was also involved in development of EURIPA, the European Rural and Isolated Practitioners Association, and I'm still executive secretary for it.[43] We've been running annual events to try to raise the profile of rural practice and rural health across Europe and we've got members from across most of Europe now. But again, it just shows you how long it takes. I think even in countries that are largely rural, people don't think they're doing anything different and anything special, and it's actually trying to get people to stand back and think about what they're doing. Interestingly, and picking up what John Hamilton says, I now work for something called Healthwatch and I run a local organization in Shropshire, which is quite a large rural county, not large in terms of Australia or Canada's geography, but large for the UK.[44] Healthwatch was set up two years ago to listen to people's voices, to their experiences of health and social care. So in Shropshire, our organization is there to do the community engagement, to go out, talk to the patients and the service users about their experiences of local health and social care.[45] We use that information to challenge the providers and the commissioners who commission those services, and pay

---

[41] The Institute of Rural Health was set up in 1997 by John Wynn-Jones and Jane Randall-Smith as a charitable foundation researching and promoting the heath of rural communities. It was closed in 2015.

[42] Rural proofing was introduced in 2000 in the Government Rural White Paper, *Our Countryside: The Future – A Fair Deal for Rural England*: Department of the Environment, Transport and the Regions (2000); for a commentary see Swindlehurst *et al*. (2005). See further discusssion on pages 62–3.

[43] See footnote 11.

[44] Healthwatch England was created following the healthcare reforms of 2012 to promote health and social care services in England through a network of branches in every local authority: www.healthwatch.co.uk/ (accessed 1 June 2016).

[45] See the Healthwatch Shropshire website at www.healthwatchshropshire.co.uk/ (accessed 23 March 2016).

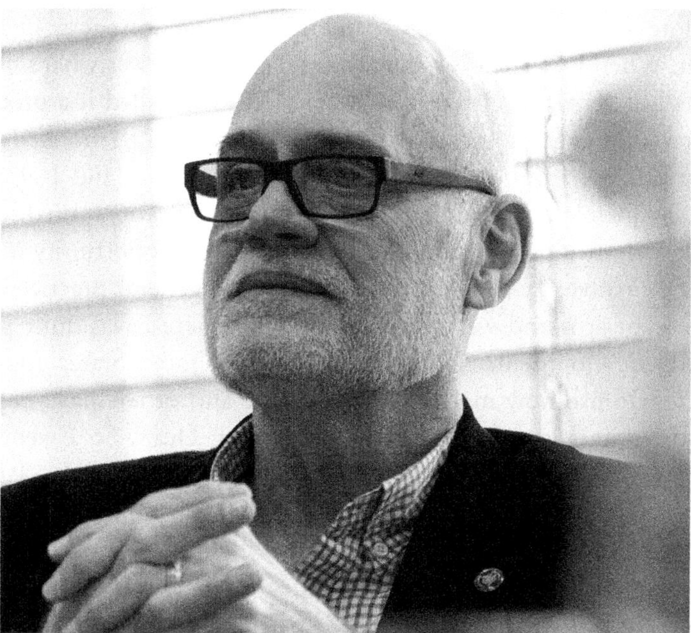

Figure 24: Professor Richard Hays

for those services. It's quite interesting how things are evolving and how much importance is now put on the consumer, if you like, because consumers have rights. We hear all the time in Shropshire that it's about access to services, it's about ambulance response times, it's about getting GP appointments, and you could almost predict the themes that are coming through because they don't really change very much month on-month or year-on-year. So, although I'm not actively involved in rural health in quite the same way I was in the Institute, we're still really involved in Shropshire because we're looking at it from the patient perspective. But that also impacts on resourcing and we're still fighting a losing battle, I think, to get effective resourcing for rural areas and for the service providers.

Roger Strasser: You mentioned Richard and Keele and now it's time to hear from Richard Hays.

Professor Richard Hays: I'm going to focus on the 1970 to 2000 period initially. I was born, raised, and educated in small communities, always wanted to be a rural GP. I had to travel 1,500 km away from home to study medicine and have had trouble getting back there on-and-off in terms of postgrad training in the early days. I was lucky in that I married somebody who is a speech pathologist, or speech language therapist, who also came from small towns, and therefore we never wanted to live in big cities. We don't actually like them very much. When I was first working in rural practice, I was what's now called a rural medical generalist, which Bruce referred to[46] I called it a proceduralist general practitioner, quite procedural in many ways. But I noticed that very few of the doctors around me were Australian graduates and I also noticed that very few people from rural and regional schools went to medical school. That stuck with me for a bit, and when I was given an opportunity in the early 1980s to be involved with vocational training for general practice and rural practice, I leapt at it and went through a phase where I was quite fascinated by the early developments, in particular in the United States and Tromsø. I've been to Tromsø now many times, and Ivar and others have been out to James Cook University where I was the founding Dean. So I went through a phase there of trying to fill in the gaps in the evidence base. I did quite a lot of early research around recruitment and retention. I was hired as the first professor of rural health in Queensland, which was an interesting move, quite controversial at the time, and then got the job as the founding Dean of James Cook University.[47] I was fascinated by how one could put together all the evidence and I described it a bit like baking a cake. You had to be creative with the recipe but there was actually some evidence somewhere around the students you selected, the kind of curriculum you put up, how you assessed, the sort of role models you presented people with, where they did placements, and how long they did rural placements. James Cook University is now almost 16 years old, it's done remarkably well, and some of you will be aware of the papers coming out.[48] There have been five publications so far, with data going up to eight years postgrad, and there are about to be more with the 10 year postgrad data. But basically the recipe is working and the cake tastes like it was intended to taste at its creation.

I think that one of the things I learned was that it's a mistake to attach medical students to rural doctors. Now this is controversial, but we went through an interesting period, just picking up on what John Hamilton said, we attached students to communities and we got the local councils and the mayors and other organizations involved. The instruction book for students included things like: play on a local sports team, go to the local hotel and have a beer, and watch the

---

[46] Page 29. See Professor Richard Hays' partly autobiographical collection of essays: Hays (2002).

[47] For the development of the James Cook University School of Medicine, see Hays (2014).

[48] See, for example, Sen Gupta *et al.* (2014); Woolley *et al.* (2014).

town work. That one got me into trouble: I had to withdraw it because students took that as a licence to go to pubs. [Laughter] But I was brought up and I had worked in many rural communities, and I knew how rural communities worked, and I wanted the students to see some of the really positive things about how small communities work.[49] I was also then really fortunate in that I got hired to come to the United Kingdom to start up Keele Medical School and that's where I came across Jane Randall-Smith. I had already met John Wynn-Jones and others as well, at that Shanghai rural medicine conference.[50] I'm quite proud of the fact that Keele, while it doesn't look innovative in the Australian context necessarily, is certainly a bit off field, out of field, in the UK and European context, with very prolonged primary care placements, half of which are in rural locations.[51] The team at Keele are fighting to maintain that despite quite a fightback from the hospital-based specialists. I haven't seen any long-term follow-up studies from Keele but I know they are coming. I am still involved with Keele, and still go there. Since that time I've branched off really, I've been involved as a consultant to many new schools around the world, some of them rural, some of them not. I've become a bit of a change leader/manager around curriculum and assessment redesign, and I'm now the Dean or Head of Programme or Head of School in my fourth medical school and, John Hamilton, I'm told it's looking like I might challenge your record. But I want to reassure you, I'm not going to try to challenge your record any further. I've really enjoyed what I've done but I sit back now and I take a lot of pleasure out of the long-term follow-up. Just to emphasize, there actually is a lot of evidence around how to do this properly, and many schools around the world are now applying that evidence. What was once very, very strange is now regarded as normal. And by strange I mean, when I was setting up James Cook University, when I had just accepted the position, the word went around the country that nobody would send their children to this medical school because any medical school run by a GP would never be able to train people who could then be in any other specialty. I was accused of training unemployable barefoot doctors, and the Deans of two metropolitan medical schools offered me chairs and money to leave North Queensland to go and set up what would be much less successful rural medicine departments, to stop the James Cook Medical

---

[49] See similar comments by Professor Richard Hays on pages 108–9.

[50] See page 11.

[51] For the curriculum at Keele University Medical School see, for example, Bartlett *et al.* (2011). See also the comments by Professor Richard Hays on Keele Medical School on pages 90 and 135–7.

School going ahead. It's hard to believe that that kind of thing went on. You weren't the chair of the committee at the time, John [Hamilton], it was a little after that time.

Roger Strasser: I think each of the introductions we've heard have highlighted some of the points that will come out in the discussion that follows. I think it's good to have these fulsome introductions because that's really going to add to the richness of the report from this Witness Seminar. I'm going to encourage moving forward and short, focused contributions to the discussion as we work our way through the topics. The first topic is the impact of specialization. I think we could have an interactive discussion around the first two topics – specialization and generalism and the relationship to rural medicine. We heard James say that in the 1970s for him at the University of Aberdeen, rural was normal. I think it is fair to say that already in all parts of the world the rather rapid development of specialization in medicine was really gaining momentum. What I call the cult of the expert, the belief that someone who has a large knowledge and a narrow field, is somehow superior to someone who has a broader knowledge in a wide field, that cult of the expert was well established in, I would say, North America and here in the UK. It was really in the early part of the twentieth century, or even before, that the momentum was there for that. But in many other parts of the world, the valuing of generalism really continued well into the latter part of the twentieth century, especially in the rural setting. Before we get to the 1970–2000 timeframe, I think we should also acknowledge the effect, not only of the development of specialization and technology in medicine, but also the impact of Abraham Flexner and his report in 1910, which set the trend for medical education since then.[52] And in particular the adherence to the concept that clinical education should take place in a teaching hospital, which by the 1970s meant acute hospitals in big cities, which were dominated by specialists and sub-specialists. So that's framing the beginning of the discussion about specialization *vis-à-vis* generalism and relationship to rural medicine.

Rourke: I want to pick up on some things both you and Richard said. Talking about Flexner, when I came back to Canada from spending time with you in Australia in 1994, I was very keen to set up a really comprehensive rural medicine programme at the University of Western Ontario and Northern Ontario, which

---

[52] The report by Abraham Flexner reviewed the state of medical education in the United States and Canada at the beginning of the twentieth century, which gave rise to far-reaching reforms and the standardization of medical education: Flexner (1910). For the impact of Flexner's report, see, for example, Duffy (2011); and see further comments by Professor John Hamilton on pages 46–7.

had a large rural area, but not remote like in parts of Canada. There was a clear need for distributed rural medical education, but I remember when the Dean and I took that to faculty council for approval, which was the highest attended faculty council there had ever been because it was contentious – and we forget how contentious these things are when we look back to this time period in the 1990s and 1980s – from the back of the room came the comment: 'Dr Rourke, you would turn us back to the pre-Flexner kind of education. Why would we ever send people out of our university hospitals for their training out in the country?' Now fortunately the Dean and I had some early preliminary data, as Richard has talked about,[53] that showed that there were some good results in rural training. When I asked the people the question: 'What was *their* data for what they were doing?' they didn't have data. And so it did proceed. But these things were controversial. Again, the impact of starting a new medical school, we encountered the same thing as Richard has said, in the Northern Ontario Medical School, where I was asked to be the chair of the original design team to come up with a blueprint that the Government could approve. But this was not on the agenda of the other medical schools who had wanted to have a colonial type approach to Northern Ontario, to the point that people were thinking that I should resign my position in the medical school I was at, because I was suggesting something counter to what would be in the interest of the traditional medical schools. This idea that medical education should be done by big tertiary care centres was the prominent theme then. The other part of that theme was the reaction of GPs to overtime. We saw in Canada, as the specialists became dominant, that GPs in the cities limited their practice. They stopped doing hospital care, they stopped delivering babies, which they had all done before, attending births. That actually worked okay in the cities. But training people for general practice in the cities no longer gave them the skills that we needed for real generalist training in the country. That's what I think founded the need to do something different, because the trend that was happening in medical education for GPs was not going to work for what we needed out in the real rural generalist kind of practice that we had in Australia and Canada. That may be different to what's needed in places like the UK, for example, but those things all tied in, the impact of specialization in the sense that tertiary care was the only place you could properly train, or the proper thing to do.

Roger Strasser: It's good we're starting in 1970 because it was in the 1970s that there was a beginning of a kind of differentiation from what's normal in, say, Aberdeen in Scotland, and I would say in Australia where the adherence

---

[53] See page 38.

to generalism really lasted into the 1970s, but then the explosion of specialties was such that new graduates from medical school from the early 1970s were all going straight into specialties. Before that they went into practice. They were general, they went into practice, and the ones who didn't do so well in practice then came back and trained to be specialists. There was a quick flip around really in the late 1960s, early 1970s, in Australia. I'm interested to hear from other parts of the world.

Douglas: My observation of the 1970s and 1980s was really that a lot of specialists, certainly within the UK, were beginning to say to those of us who were doing things like delivering babies, even if we hadn't had any problems doing that, that we shouldn't be doing this sort of thing, this was the province of the specialist, so specialists were empire-building. There were also other professional groups like midwives saying: 'We want to do that. We don't want GPs involved.' So there was a lot of stuff behind the scenes, a lot of health service politics, I suppose. And we were beginning to get the things that we'd learned how to do taken away from us. Just take a very simple example like the insertion of coils for contraception: there then became a movement, a specialty was developing by the Faculty of Reproductive Health in the UK, and people would then come along and say: 'Well, unless you're doing 12 of these a month or something like that, then you're not competent at doing it. Show us your records to say that you're still competent,' etc. So the whole question and the fear and the threat, even if something hadn't actually happened, there were lots of peer threats about litigation and so on, what would happen if this went wrong? How have you been trained? What is your accreditation? These sorts of things. So the march of the specialists is quite a complex thing, but lots of things had been taken away from generalists by those marching specialists wanting to outline their area of turf. That's fair enough in a city but it doesn't fit with trying to provide a service in a rural area.

Roger Strasser: We're talking so far about developed countries. I'm interested to get a sense of what was happening around that time in developing countries, say in South Africa. Ian Couper?

Couper: The divide has been substantial in South Africa certainly, but I think for a lot of Africa it hasn't been so much a general practice versus specialist divide, as an urban hospital versus rural hospital divide. Most of healthcare until probably the last two decades or so, has been provided out of hospitals where doctors have been involved in rural areas in Africa. One of the things I was reflecting on when Richard Hays was talking about barefoot doctors etc.,[54] was that's what I've been accused of doing in terms of training mid-level workers. In Africa mid-level workers have played a major role in rural healthcare. So some of the debate, rather than specialist versus generalist, has been: should it be doctors or should it be other levels of workers who are providing the care and the services? Many countries in Africa depend on medical assistants, clinical officers, *technicos* – they're called different things in different countries – to provide most of the rural care.[55] If you go to places like Malawi, Tanzania, Uganda, you will find hospitals that are fully run by clinical officers, who have a large amount of experience, and very often without doctors. Or, one place I went to, which was a regional hospital in Malawi, there were specialists and there were clinical officers; and the specialists, who were overseas-trained specialists, didn't know what to do because they didn't have the interns and junior doctors to work with them. So there was a complete disconnect and dysfunctionality in the hospital because they didn't understand how to fit into a system that worked differently. In fact, in terms of specialists in rural hospitals, we went through that with the Cuban doctor programme in South Africa where we had Cuban specialists coming into our rural hospitals who were trained as specialists and they would not have the support they needed.[56] So a typical example would be an obstetrician coming into a rural district hospital who couldn't do Caesarean sections because there was no anaesthetist, and they would not be prepared to learn anaesthetics because their registration and everything was around the fact that they were obstetricians. It was only as the people involved in the programme came to understand that you need a generalist family physician in the rural hospital, and that the specialists are much better in a regional or bigger hospital, that that started to change. So I think that's been a major factor in the way that the services have been run. I think it's interesting in terms of the history of health professions, education, and rural medical education that the mid-level worker in Africa has been completely left out of that process of modernization.[57] If we get frustrated with the way medical education happens, to see how some of these training programmes are within ministries of health and have been running programmes that were established in the 1970s and have never changed – their teaching methods haven't changed and their content

---

[54] See page 39.

[55] For a review of mid-level health workers see, for example, Lehmann (2008).

[56] For the Cuban doctor programme see, for example, Hammett (2007).

[57] Doherty *et al.* (2013).

hasn't changed; it gives you an idea of some of the challenges. These people are often trained to be in positions for which there is no career pathway, no career ladder. So it's a dead end but it does provide an opportunity for training. Many people then go and do other things or go into illegal private practice, etc. So I think that's an interesting additional dimension to rural practice in Africa.[58]

Roger Strasser: I'm wondering, Maja, if you have any observations on these issues from your perspective?

Račić: Well, it's a little hard to comment because the circumstances in which we work in Bosnia are a bit different when you compare it to Canada, or to the United States, or to South Africa. Actually we have one programme in family medicine and through that programme we are trying to get our residents to spend a part of their training in a rural region. So, for example, 18 months of their training they do here in Foča, in the rural hospital, and the other 18 months they spend in the Family Medicine Education Centre (and, of those, several months are spent in a rural clinic). I think it's very important because many of our doctors are working in rural regions and so their needs are different to the needs of urban doctors, especially in the regions where the nearest hospital is very far away. So they need to have a greater variety of skills than the doctors working in urban regions. The main problem here is that our Ministry of Health has a completely different attitude to rural doctors and urban doctors, and it's really hard to work in a rural region because of the payment system and because rural doctors have to do a lot of services they are not paid for. But actually they have to do it and we have to prepare people for that. I think in rural medicine they can do better family medicine than in the towns and cities in Bosnia Herzegovina, so the residency is very important. Since we have different circumstances we need to make changes through the family medicine residency programme, the only one that we have within the country.[59]

Roger Strasser: That's a very helpful comment and my mind connects to Ian Couper mentioning the doctors from Cuba. Of course, during this period, the Soviet era, the cult of specialism had gone to the full extreme in Russia and related countries where, right from the beginning of medical school, they were trained to become a specialist. Of course, that then affected the whole structure

---

[58] For a review of rural healthcare in sub-Saharan Africa see, for example, Strasser, Kam, and Regalado (2016).

[59] See Račić (2015).

of the system and the priorities for resourcing as well. John Hamilton, you've lived and worked in many parts of the world, including Africa and Asia, and the private practice bit that Ian mentioned reminds me that in Thailand the programme they have to support and encourage rural practice there includes paying what's called a 'laziness bonus' – that is to encourage the rural doctors not to have a private practice but to have a sufficient reward for providing care in the public system in the rural communities in Thailand.[60] So would you like to share your observations from the various countries you've been in, John?

Hamilton: Well, thank you. Just on Thailand: I did a review there when I was part of the World Bank and at that time they'd put some very constructive things in place to get doctors into rural areas. They had done away with the system that you didn't get into training if you ever left the teaching hospital. They changed it that you couldn't get into advanced training unless you'd gone into rural hospitals. They took away the salary ceiling that was put on rural practitioners so that they could rise both in seniority and salary as well as the specialty doctors, so there was quite a lot of structural change at that time to encourage it.[61] If I pick out the theme of the barefoot doctors: in 1978 when we set Ilorin up, I had nine months to get the curriculum going and didn't even have somewhere to live for that time. A lot of people said, well, some of the rather snooty academics – and there were many that were not snooty and very good, around about in other schools – said: 'You're just doing barefoot doctors because you're going into the village.' So the barefoot doctor was flung at our head and, going back 30, 40 years later, it's still going on and the university is getting all of its faculties to go out into the communities. That's very much like the social accountability of universities as a whole. I've also been working with the big teaching hospital in Lagos College of Medicine helping them with some reforms and Victor [Inem] has been involved in that. I was very pleased to find that the Ilorin graduates, when they go down as interns, and now some are consultants, are seen as very good clinicians. So they have a good public health perspective and they have a very good clinician perspective.

---

[60] For rural healthcare in Thailand see, for example, Wibulpolprasert and Pengpaiboon (2003).

[61] Professor John Hamilton wrote: 'The steps taken by the Ministry of Health were to: equalise between rural and urban employment (previously disadvantageous to rural); requirement for rural service prior to advanced postgraduate training; the ceiling for advancement in rural employment raised to the full height, reserved previously only for specialists in metropolitan employment.' Email to Ms Caroline Overy, 27 June 2016.

Now, if you go to other countries, I've been going into Iran the last few years and they are doing some interesting reforms in medical education.[62] When I was first there, before the revolution, they were introducing a strong programme of village health workers, which is for rural areas and widely distributed. I've had a look at that again: they've got better vaccination success than Australia has; they have been tracking nutrition of children and they have arrangements in clusters with doctors coming in and out, but the village health workers come from the village and they live there, and they're well trained. There's an interesting transition about to happen: they have for some time been thinking that neither undergraduate education is prepared for family medicine nor is there any real constructive training or career structure – they are strongly considering introducing family medicine, and the papers I've got in draft do not mention this village health worker system. Now that might be very dangerous to expect that medical doctors will take over the role successfully done by the village health workers. Amanda Howe, who I think is WONCA president now, has just been to Iran to advise. So WONCA is probably going to have quite a hand in that, but it's very tricky if the name 'family medicine' – and many people that I've talked to didn't really know what it meant – is seen as the doctors making a bold step forward and in danger of dislodging a system that's been providing very good preferable, rural care. Very tricky that.

Can I have two minutes to say something about Flexner?[63] What Flexner was opposing in the small country towns was a lot of practitioners setting up cheap dash-and-run medical schools that, even though they had accrediting jurisdictions, nobody would apply to them. There was no scientific base, no satisfactory organization of teaching, that's what he was opposing. He was taking the German example and putting emphasis on science, not as detailed knowledge but as a way of thinking, the logic, what we would call now actually learning by discovery and the hypothetico-deductive process. He was asked whether this was necessary for those who were going to work in rural areas, and surely they didn't need all this. And he said that, actually, they needed it even more because they didn't have people to turn to, and every step in their experience was going to be an education for them to build their inside sum knowledge. He also said that his plan of action should not go forever, it should be reviewed in 20 years when times are different. Nobody reviewed that really up until this time. Various somewhat educationally illiterate commissions have

---

[62] Hamilton (2011).

[63] See pages 40–1 and note 52.

written big papers and flown around the world, but people just carried things on. He was really describing problem-based learning, learning by enquiry, getting into the community just like getting into the wards. I feel quite defensive about Flexner because very few people have actually read him.

Roger Strasser: I agree with what you're saying about what Flexner said and what he intended; it's not actually what happened and how others interpreted what he said, let alone developments that he couldn't have imagined from when he delivered his report.

Douglas: Just really coming back to the topic impact of specialization in the time period 1970–2000. One of the things that we've seen during that time period is really the change, certainly in the UK, in the role of women in medicine and women within society – the generation that are currently going to be, or aspiring to be, doctors, or are young doctors, and the whole thing about Generation Y. So we now in the UK have, it is correct and good that this is so, a greater proportion of women in medicine than we have men. One of the impacts of that is the attractiveness of specialization. It is 'quite easy' to be a specialist today. If you are a cardiologist you are either an electrician or a plumber to the heart. If you're a young woman with children, it's a very easy choice to make to decide to be an electrician for the heart or a plumber for the heart. And one of the difficulties we have, the two specialties within the UK that are finding it really difficult to recruit, are the two big generalist things – nobody wants to be an A&E doctor in the UK, nobody wants to be a general practitioner in the UK. Those are the two generalist specialties, and I think many of the Generation Y people, the people who have been brought up during this time period from 1970 to 2000, have different, or changing, cultural values which we can debate at length. But that is another direct impact of how specialization, through the cultural things that have occurred in that time period, is now impacting on medicine today.

Sarah Strasser: I just wanted to comment that I've had an opportunity recently to reread some of Donald Schön's work, which was in the 1970s and 1980s.[64] I found it very interesting to compare what he was writing about at the time, which was a concern of overspecialization in society to our current issues with

---

[64] Donald Schön (1930–1997) was a philosopher and Ford Professor of Urban Studies and Education at MIT. His works include *Technology and Change: The new Heraclitus* (1967); *The Reflective Practitioner. How professionals think in action* (1983); and *Beyond the Stable State. Public and private learning in a changing society* (1971), which followed his Reith Lectures 'Change and Industrial Society' given in 1970.

overspecialization. He pointed out that it was difficult, at that time, to even get oneself breakfast without relying on technology and that there was a specialist approach to every single bit of getting breakfast and it was a specialist design to breakfast. I think it's interesting that we have taken on board what's happening in society more generally and the issue of commodification of everything is worrisome, yet in many ways there are aspects that are improving so we've got to capture those bits. It strikes me that one of the special areas of rural medicine is the communication and connections and networking that we make, which you have to have to compensate for all this commodification. I don't know what the answer is but I thought there were some linkages there worth raising.

Roger Strasser: Donald Schön was at the Massachusetts Institute of Technology, so you might say in Boston they're leading the world in terms of that kind of technological development. But what he wrote about was reflection in action understanding and know-how type knowledge, which is, I think, central to rural practice.

Hays: Just a brief comment. Nobody's brought this up so far, but, in fact, the response of us, and many of our colleagues, was to make general practice and rural practice specialties. So we, in a sense, were forced to go down the same route and, since 2000 – with, as we have defined, more proceduralist specialist rural doctors – we have been splitting them up into little sub-specialty roles. So, for instance, the kind of proceduralist I was – I was primarily a procedural obstetrician and surgeon but I could give a very safe back-up general anaesthetic and do a lot of regional anaesthesia. It's very rare in Australia now to find somebody who would do anaesthetics and other procedures whereas 30–40 years ago it was the norm. So, I think we have been both part of the specialization process, which initially was very helpful, more recently maybe less so.

Sarah Strasser: I have a metaphor that in the 1980s when I moved to Australia and we went to buy our washing machine my natural inclination was to go to the city and look at all the available models. I then went back to our hometown and discovered that basically there were only two available locally and only one would be serviced in our house. So the choice was zero.

Roger Strasser: That's a generalist washing machine.

Wynn-Jones: I think there's another element in this, Roger. We went through a period of specialization and a de-skilling of general practitioners a lot earlier than many places did, and I think this is the same in Europe. By the 1970s we didn't have many procedural GPs left. We had GPs who were doing obstetrics, but the obstetrics was lost to midwives. One of my anxieties is that this has put small hospitals at risk. There is a need to establish essential district general hospitals in rural areas staffed by generalists. I am aware that the Scots have got the same problem. It's actually very difficult now to attract generalist surgeons, general physicians to these hospitals, as we've already seen in West Wales with the reduction of services in these hospitals becoming unviable. There's a hospital in Aberystwyth, which is right on the western fringe of Wales (on the coast), and they used to be able to attract ex-army doctors who were still generalists, but those are now drying up as the army is reducing its military medical capacity. We have a situation in Aberystwyth, where women in labour, unless they're seen as being no-risk cases, now have to go another hour and a half and be transferred in labour to Carmarthen, which is a considerable way away. It's not only that we are losing services but we're actually endangering small hospitals by the growth and the speed of the specialist revolution.

Roger Strasser: I think that's a very important comment. I'm aware that, in terms of going through the set topics, we're still only on the second point, although I think we've touched on others (see the Outline Programme on page 8). I'm certainly going to encourage keeping moving, and also looking ahead to future topics if you want to make those connections when you are speaking. We could have a four-hour seminar on each one of these topics but we're not going to. So, before we get back into the discussion of the topics, I'd like to give the opportunity to the people who have recently joined us on the video link to introduce themselves.

Professor Victor Inem: I'm really by heart a rural practitioner in Nigeria. I've practised at Pakoto and also in Itigidi and Abakaliki. I am a professor of family medicine with a lot of emphasis in the area of rural health. I've been involved since the 1980s in the development of family medicine and rural health and primary healthcare in Nigeria. I want to say something quickly about what John Hamilton said about community health workers – that for us we have to see doctors who venture to work in rural areas as true philanthropists, in that they should see physicians or doctors who come into the rural areas as consultants to the process as opposed to real service providers. Because once they see us as a service provider they see us as competitors. But when you come as a consultant, as a facilitator to the process, there's a chance to be considered partners, and a lot of community health workers tend to want to work with you. Through that you can then give them a lot of training. In family medicine we have

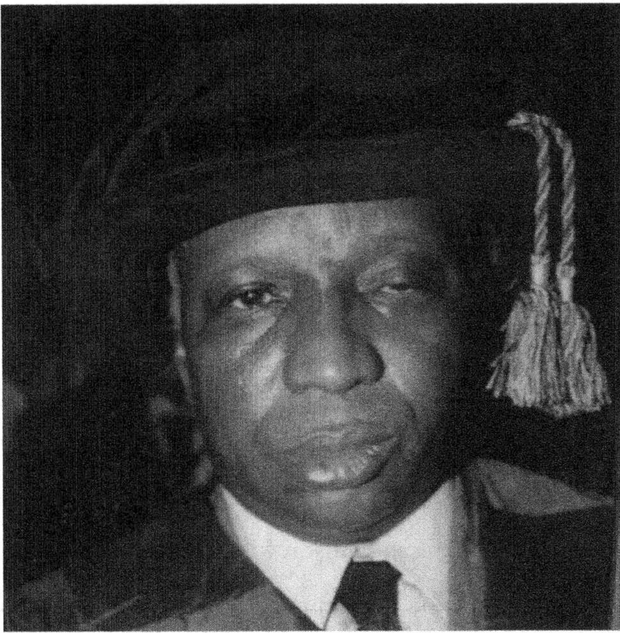

Figure 25: Professor Victor Inem

concentrated more using faith-based hospitals and community hospitals based in rural settings as training centres for our resident doctors in family medicine and the community health officers.

Dr Oleg Kravtchenko: I'm a rural GP and a mentor practising in coastal northern Norway, between Tromsø and Trondheim for 10 plus years. For me the development of rural medicine and medicine generally in recent years from 1970 to 2000 looks like it follows this pendulum route where it moves from generalized to sub-specialization and then perhaps will move back, and then hopefully will balance in the middle. I guess some countries, because of territorial peculiarities or perhaps the education pattern, they cut this natural generalism in this stage; such countries such as Australia, United States, and Europe, especially Spain and Norway and Sweden as well. I guess this development will proceed in the same direction.

Roger Strasser: We're going to continue working our way through the outline programme but I want to connect them and try to make sure we cover something about all of them as we go. A theme that I think we'll come back to is about the relationship with the community. Several of you, as you introduced yourselves, talked about the importance for students, in particular, to be immersed in a community and learn from the community, not just be

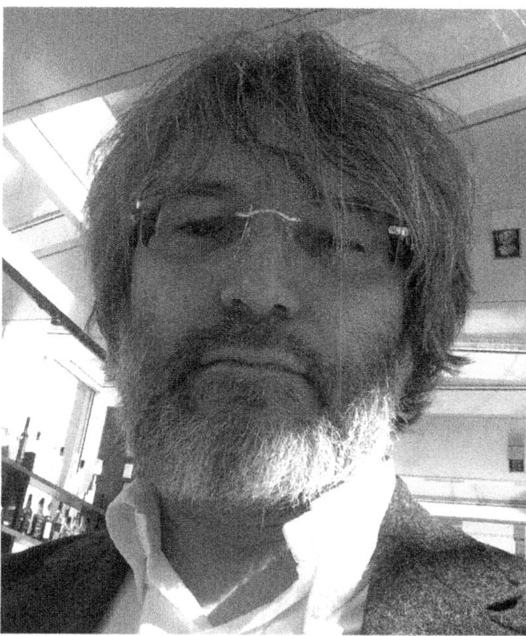
Figure 26: Dr Oleg Kravtchenko

attached to a doctor. And, of course, part of rural medicine is that the doctor is part of the community, lives in the community, and is acutely aware, and so the focus of rural medicine is responding to community need. But at the same time, as we described, the development of specialization has created a hierarchy within the medical profession, with the sub-specialists in the big city teaching hospital at the top and, I guess, the general practitioners and family physicians somewhere near the bottom, and rural practitioners don't even qualify to be in the hierarchy. That's the way it is for the medical profession. We heard the slur of being accused of being a barefoot doctor – that's even worse really, when you think about it. Yet in the communities themselves the status of the rural practitioner is very high, and that's the sort of dimension that we need to note.

We started touching on the technological developments and transportation and communication. John Wynn-Jones commented about Aberystwyth and now travelling for services. I would say during that period, 1970–2000, there were phases where governments were, shall we say, sold or bought into the idea that technology, both communication technology and information technology and transportation technology, meant that there didn't have to be the full range of services in remote and rural communities, because, with the telemedicine, you don't need rural doctors, you just need telemedicine, because the flying squad can come in and pick up the sick person and transport them back to the city where they'll get the high-class specialist treatment. So that idea was there, but it didn't exactly work out that way, and maybe that's a good jumping off point to pick up on the impact of technological developments and move forward in our list of topics.

We might come back to national/international networks a little later, but can we connect this to the relationship with other health professionals? Victor talked about the health workers, mid-levels, as part of the team rather than competition. I would say living in rural communities all of the health workers are acutely aware of the needs and tend to work together to address those needs because they're part of the community, because that's part of being a rural practitioner.

Douglas: During this period of 1970–2000 I think the impact of technology has been significant. Certainly in my own practice I started, or we started, without computers, and during this time personal computers were invented and became available to all. So, certainly, I can remember a period in my own practice where we started off with the most basic computers in the UK at that time, BBC Acorn computers and so on, to build up age/sex registers. Now we're at the stage, that revolution has continued and certainly in the UK, where we have a list-based system for patients, we code people for what they come to see us with that day and what medicines we've given them and what diseases they've got. The whole thing is about micro-epidemiology – so at a click of a button today, and even as far back as 2000, I could tell you how many people have had heart attacks in my practice, or how many people are on which drug, or whatever. I think that's been one of the huge benefits of technology in rural practice, and rural doctors have adopted that. Rural doctors have been early adopters of technology, certainly computing technology. The other thing that's had an influence on our practice is just the organization. We've been talking about specialist care, we can think of numerous technical innovations that have occurred in wider medicine, so, for instance, in cardiology the introduction of stents and angioplasty and things like that have required us in rural practice to make sure that we organize our care for early identification of what might be wrong with somebody. So in times gone by, certainly in the early stages of the 1970s in a rural practice, we might have tucked up somebody in bed at home, as I remember doing in my early stages of general practice, with a heart attack. Now that would never be seen to be so. We instantly have to get somebody whisked away to a centre in a city to get angioplasty or stents or whatever.

So, certainly, the impacts of technology and medical technology have changed, and the impacts of new patient testing are another technology that have been universally applied in rural practice as well as wider urban practice – just simple things like people knowing their blood sugars and their own blood pressure, or whatever. All these things have had a big impact and improvement in healthcare and health outcomes in rural practice. So technology has definitely helped this.

Roger Strasser: Well, I'm seeing it more as a mixed picture but let's leave it at that.

Rourke: I want to pick up on some comments that you said about the hierarchy, professional identity, and technology and see if I can put it all together. I think one of the most fundamental things that happened in the period 1970–2000, particularly in the late 1980s and 1990s, was the regrasping of the professional identity of the rural doctor. So with this hierarchy – general practice at the bottom and rural practice somewhere outside, not even seen by many people as relevant anymore – what started happening (led by Australia, the Rural Doctors Association of Australia, like Bruce Chater talked about, Ian Couper in South Africa, the Society of Rural Physicians in Canada) had a profound impact bringing world doctors together, not as part of general practice, where they were dominated by city meetings, but part of their own meetings and groups and developing their own identity and own support network. In fact, that was helped by the technology of the fax machine, which allowed us to communicate around the world very quickly before we could actually have the internet to do that. Professional identity was suffering, and it was those groups that really brought the support and identity back to make rural practice into something strong and unique that needs to be strived for. The foundation that drove that was bringing people together with the common goal of providing access to care to a population that was not getting access to care, and that challenge is still going on today. As John Wynn-Jones says, access is the number one issue in rural practice. Part of the identity of rural doctors is that most rural doctors are in it because it's more of a calling than a career opportunity – they're trying to respond to the needs of their communities, rather than trying to offer a refined set of skills that is a career not a calling. So it's more responding to the needs of the community as their identity, as opposed to providing a specific service that can be limited.

Roger Strasser: Thanks, Jim. I said we'd skip over national and international organizations but you hit the mark really well, of the value of national organizations and the international connections, in talking about the rural doctor organizations that formed in the 1980s and the 1990s. Of course, the

WONCA Working Party we've mentioned, but there are other opportunities where rural doctors have connected across national borders and found they have more in common with each other than they have with their colleagues in their own field in the big cities. I think that's certainly a theme that we need to recognize in terms of identity and the value of those networks. I'm keen to hear comments from others on the developing themes here.

Wynn-Jones: Just some of my experience from an international perspective on setting up networks: I was able, with Jane and some colleagues across Europe, to set up EURIPA.[65] We really had a 15-year struggle to get it recognized. So it's not just the specialists who are against us but our own colleagues. WONCA Europe was originally established from three networks: the research network, the education network, and the quality network. They wouldn't allow us to engage. Our own profession, our own discipline, sometimes actually stands in our way more than anything else. We were not seen as scientific, we were not seen as credible educationalists, and that's been a real struggle. I suspect that you'll find that in other parts of the world as well.

Couper: That's right. I want to pick up on the network and technology but then move back to something that Victor was talking about. In the rural hospital that I worked in, in the 1970s and early 1980s, prior to my being there, they connected by shortwave radio. The four hospitals in the area had a weekly journal club on two-way radio, so they were using technology in that way. Then in the 1990s the development of email was an incredible advance for us in terms of being able to connect, and we started a mailing list for all doctors, where we could share clinical problems and get help, because too often one couldn't get that help from specialists. They weren't really interested in providing that help and it was our rural colleagues that provided the clinical help. It's interesting that mostly rural doctors now don't feel the need for that anymore because there are generally more doctors in each site to provide that assistance, and there's also more support from specialists that there didn't used to be.

I want to pick up on something that Victor mentioned, and it comes back to one of the things I was talking about. Victor was mentioning the role of the church hospitals, the mission hospitals, in Africa. I think that one of the fascinating things in the history of Africa is the role of missions in rural Africa because, as the decolonization occurred in the 1960s and 1970s, the colonial powers withdrew, and in many cases they left very little behind. In many

---

[65] See note 11.

countries, with some exceptions, they had failed to develop good educational systems, proper training systems, etc. So there was a deficit and often it was the mission hospitals, certainly in rural areas outside the cities, that were carrying that forward. They continued to be a major part of healthcare, particularly rural healthcare, in Africa in different ways. In South Africa it was slightly different because of apartheid – the mission hospitals were there but missionaries were suspected by the regime of working with communities against the regime, and again close working with the community in a rural hospital was key. So the apartheid regime actually made it very uncomfortable for missions to continue. They stopped providing funding, they made it difficult for mission doctors to come, etc., and the majority of mission hospitals actually handed over their facilities to governments, to the South African Government and to the Homeland so-called independent states that existed. Some of the hospitals that managed to continue, even though they were government hospitals, continued with a kind of mission ethos in terms of the way they functioned – not necessarily in terms of the religious component but their networking with the community and the broader perspective, rather than just the purely medical – and were some of those that really continued to be very strong and have a major impact.

The last thing I want to say related to that goes back further than the 1970s but actually has an impact to today. That is that two pioneers, in what is essentially rural health, were Sidney and Emily Kark in the 1940s in South Africa, who set up the Pholela Health Centre, which was the foundation of community-oriented primary care.[66] That was to be the first of a whole network of community health centres that were stopped not long after the National Party came to power in South Africa in 1948. Sidney and Emily Kark emigrated to Israel and developed community-orientated primary care in Israel and from there it was exported to the USA, to Brazil, to Cuba, to many other parts of the world. And it's finally, in the last 10 years or so, arriving back in South Africa and we've been revisiting what they did and re-establishing that. Some of that is around what Victor and others have been talking about, that working together with community health workers, that teamwork across different professional levels, which has been a very interesting process to watch.

Hamilton: What Ian was just saying: the challenge to the apartheid regime was that they were working with, and empowering, the community and that is very, very much resented by any dominant group. Now, I have a very strong sense that students and individuals benefit a lot, not only from networks, but

---

[66] See Tollman (1994).

individual exploration of issues in other settings. Sandy Eades, who was one of our first Aboriginal graduates, and is now Professor of Indigenous Health, was a very shy girl when she started.[67] Her biggest eye-opening experience was to go first to Bangladesh as a student and see other communities detached from the somewhat introspective problems of the indigenous settings, overcoming troubles, and then working with the first Mohawk doctor who qualified in Canada. She saw that leadership could be hers and that transformed the way she looked. When we finally had an indigenous conference, out of which planning came the Australian Indigenous Doctors Association (AIDA),[68] and numbers of other things, all of us who were not indigenous got out of the way; they had invited numbers of North American indigenous doctors and students, 20–30 years ahead of Australia in political progress, legal, health, all sorts of settings, and that gave them a fresh sense of independence in thinking about it. They were no longer constrained only to think from the Australian perspective. I'm going to be sending people, I hope, to New Mexico, where they're opening up the notion of other health providers because they found that the doctors were not being seen by rural people as close to them. Who did they like best? The agricultural extension officers.[69] So they're setting up that new stream. If you go back to the early nineteenth century when America was looking at how to train its public health workers, what they said was: 'The best thing to do is to look at the agricultural health extension officers, and train a group like that.' So what goes round, comes round. But go to another place, open your mind from your own preoccupations and you'll come back with a different set of views.

Aaraas: Thank you for bringing up all those themes, which have stimulated fruitful thoughts and many interesting comments. I would like to make a comment from Norway about the relationship to other health professionals and the contribution of the decentralized health education model of the Medical School in Tromsø on that theme. From the outset, it was a priority to focus on doctors and their role without giving much attention to the relationships with other health professionals. However, the year away from campus with placement in local hospitals and rural areas inevitably led medical students to interact with

---

[67] Professor Sandra Eades is the Head of Indigenous Maternal and Child Health and Associate Head of Preventative Health Research, at the Baker IDI Heart & Diabetes Institute, Melbourne.

[68] AIDA was established in 1997 following a conference at Salamander Bay in New South Wales. For the history of the organization see their website at www.aida.org.au/about-us/our-history/ (accessed 11 April 2016).

[69] See, for example, Kaufman *et al.* (2010).

other professionals. In addition, and parallel with the decentralized education for medical students, there has been an invention of similar decentralized education models for a series of health professional disciplines in Northern Norway. Initially, this was introduced as a kind of crisis intervention. Rural-living persons who wanted to contribute to improve local healthcare (as nurses, health-assistants, etc.) were admitted into education groups based on individual training and learning in their own communities, alternating with joint sessions at the organizing school. These programmes were popular and successful and turned out to be a permanent solution to recruit competent and educated health professionals to underprivileged rural communities.[70] The success of decentralized medical and health professional education models in Northern Norway from 1970 up to 2000 is well described in two Norwegian books. A problem about countries like Norway is that we are not English-speaking and publish books in our own language, inaccessible for most international readers. However, these two books document this kind of decentralized education in an interesting way from two perspectives: the perspective of educating doctors and that of educating other health professionals.[71] I think this development in Northern Norway, where I have spent my professional life, has had an important impact on the transformation of the original Faculty of Medicine at the University of Tromsø into the present Faculty of Health Sciences. Today, the faculty includes eight health professional disciplines brought together in the same premises, very much broadened from the original focus on education of doctors alone. Increasingly, students from various health professions are together in joint educational activities, both at campus and during placement periods in rural areas. I think the rising activity of student interaction learning we see today is promising. I regard this to be a fruit of the successful educational inventions described, which happened in Northern Norway during the period 1970–2000.

Roger Strasser: That's a theme really of learning in communities and clinical settings where you expect the graduates to practise in the future, and of interprofessional education as well.

Sarah Strasser: I just wanted to pick up on the point that Ivar has just made in that, interestingly, reflecting what works and what doesn't work in rural practice, in Canada a huge amount of money from the Government was effectively

---

[70] See Aaraas, Halvorsen, and Aasland (2015).

[71] Gamnes and Rasmussen (eds) (2013); Jensen (2008).

dumped into interprofessional education. When the money dried up, so did the interprofessional education. It is now minimal compared to what it was at its peak. I was just thinking that is exactly the same as what happens with rural recruitment and retention – if you give them the financial incentive and the programme runs, it only goes for as long as the money.

Roger Strasser: Yes, and part of that is, of course, the gravy train effect that suddenly urban academic institutions discover rural when they think there's money in rural; and the money dries up and their interest dries up. The same with the technology, the technological enthusiasts persuade government, if you invest in telemedicine so that everyone is into telemedicine, and so it goes on.

Inem: Well, it is the changing pattern of rurality since 1970. You just wake up one morning, you are in the midst of the big forest and the next morning you wake up, you find that the whole town has come to you. This is happening so rapidly that sometimes the rural community is not able to respond adequately and effectively to the changes that come in. Usually it's really the rural doctor that gives leadership in this area as to the type of technologies, the new concepts in diagnosis, treatment that now comes into the area, so you find that a place that was fully rural ends up being very periurban or suburban, becomes urban in the 30 years between 1970 and 2000. So we have found that a lot of what we are doing in primary healthcare in the direct rural areas we have to be tweaking it and changing a few things just to accommodate the new realities that have occurred in the environment.

Roger Strasser: Well, thanks, Victor. I think you've picked up on a couple of important things: one is the rapidity of change, the momentum really was picking up in that 30-year period. The other is the urbanization of the world. I think it was about 2009 when the tipping point came that the majority of the people in the world are now in the cities rather than in rural areas. But still almost 50 per cent of people are living in rural areas.[72] There is that assumption they have in the cities that really the solution is for everybody to move to the cities – then we wouldn't have any issues about rural health and rural health services and so on. M K Rajakumar from Malaysia, who was a former president of WONCA and member of the Working Party on Rural Practice, was a great philosopher and his view was that actually it's in our

---

[72] In 2006, 49.6 per cent of the world's population was classed as urban; in 2007 it had risen to 50.1 per cent; in 2009, it was 51.1 per cent and in 2015 it was 54 per cent. See the United Nations, Department of Economic and Social Affairs Population Division website at http://esa.un.org/unpd/wup/ (accessed 6 June 2016).

genes, living in the forest in the countryside, is what feels right.[73] It's natural to be here in part of the broader environment, and cities are only just the last few centuries, a very recent phenomenon. That's why people from cities somehow feel more comfortable and relaxed out in the rural environment. I don't know about that but I think we've picked up on some things already about the rural/ urban divide issues in terms of hospitals, in terms of service capabilities, and in terms of the assumption that we find in the cities, that anything that happens outside the cities is by definition second class or of a lesser standard. By my reckoning we've at least touched on something like seven of the eleven topics in our suggested programme and so I'll encourage people who haven't spoken to speak up and I'll use a kind of roll call approach as well. It's been quite unusual not to hear from Bruce Chater, so, if you're still awake, Bruce, I'm sure you have a lot to say about all of these themes.

Chater: Thanks, Roger. It's been very interesting hearing people's contributions and I'd just like to make a couple of comments. I think basically in the 1990s, if you look at what's been called the rural/urban divide, it was really about us pulling up the drawbridge at that stage, because we felt in rural medicine that a lot of the skills, the activities, were being given away to specialists in urban areas. I think that we were a fair distance away from the centres, particularly in Australia, and we could pull up the drawbridge a little bit. It was a bit of a defensive move back in those times. That continued on into 2000 and the early 2000s, and I don't want to take us beyond the time that you've set, but I think it is changing now. Technology, which was starting to happen in the 1990s and 2000s, is now allowing us to keep ourselves better educated, have point-of-care testing, have other technologies in rural areas, and is allowing us to work up patients a lot better. The cities and the specialists in the cities, are increasingly having patients in hospital for a very short time and so we're moving back towards, I think, rural doctors being able to actually build up the picture of their patients fairly well, send them off to the cities briefly, and bring them back again. There is the potential there for a renaissance, and that potential really started with the technology of internet, email and teleconference, video conference, and those sort of things that really had its roots in the late 1990s. Richard's touched on the identity of rural medicine and the decentralized education, and that's helping us a lot and that is another trend that started in the 1990s.

---

[73] Dr M K Rajakumar (1932–2008) was a Malaysian socialist politician and doctor, and proponent of family medicine. He was President of WONCA from 1986 to 1989. See Leng (2011).

I just want to touch on one thing that troubles me these days and it's not really on the agenda but it's happened over this time, and that is that patients have been seen increasingly as something that's out there that comes and sees you from a distance, and you shouldn't actually be able to know your patients. There's this feeling that if you know your patients, you're too close to them; for rural doctors that's the opposite of what we do. We pride ourselves on knowing our patients and being aware of our patients and their needs. In the cities, I think, there's this tendency towards them being pushed away. In fact, if you do know your patients well then there might be some almost conflict of interest or lack of judgement. I think it's a disturbing trend for rural doctors but there seems to be this common theme coming through in medicine from the cities now. I would like to hear from others so I'll leave it just there.

Roger Strasser: It's a good comment, thanks Bruce. This idea that doctors should have no relationship with their patients other than the doctor–patient or patient–doctor relationship, and of course when you live in a rural community as a rural doctor, it's impossible not to have relationships – you have to go and buy things at the shop and you have a whole life outside of being a doctor. So a very important point.

Pekez-Pavlisko: I would like to say first that technology has already helped us a lot in networking. Before the internet it was very difficult to make good networks, and I'm very thankful to John [Wynn-Jones] that he established EURIPA and ran it when it was the hardest time, when you couldn't use the internet. Rural physicians weren't in universities and it was very difficult to pick up people in different parts of Europe, or across the world, to be together. So I think technology is our power at this moment. Secondly, what I would say is, think about the pharmaceutical industry making hospital specialists gods and putting us in backstage, for example, because we weren't so interesting for the pharmaceutical industry we couldn't make good studies for them. Thirdly, what I want to give on the plate, is the situation of physicians in south-east Europe. I can tell you that in the former Yugoslavia we had a very good health system. All citizens had insurance, health insurance, they didn't have waiting lists for hospitalization and so on. After transition it hasn't been so good because politicians wanted to change everything. There was nothing good in the former system and they wanted to change everything – even good things. Now we, and all of south-east Europe, have some problems regarding the organization of all the health system and especially of rural medicine. It's a problem that we don't have enough time for lobbying the politicians. The majority of our politicians think we are not good enough when we are rural physicians. That is all from me at this moment.

Roger Strasser: So a specialist is god and we are backstage, and then the ebb and flow that goes with changing regime from a political point of view will affect the dynamics, I suppose, of rural health and rural practice.

Hays: About professional status and its implication for medical education: one of the things that bothered me as a student and as an academic in the early days is that most of the examples presented to medical students about rural medicine were negative. It was all about the big hospital rescuing this poor, rural individual who had never been able to be sorted out by some poor old clumsy but well-intentioned rural doctor. I've written a bit about this in some of the education journals and some of you may have read it.[74] One of the things I've always tried to do wherever I've worked is to put in some reverse examples because there are some. I've also made sure that we present students with cases, through PBL (problem-based learning) cases and CBL (case-based learning) cases, and general teaching, as well as immersion in practice, really good examples of practice with great outcomes for patients. I don't need to tell the audience today that there's a lot of that. So it's just one of those things that when you have a curriculum written by urban-based specialists, they base their teaching on what they've seen. And they see a different population with different prior probabilities and sometimes a long track record of things not being quite worked out. What they don't see is all the amazingly good stuff that happens in general practice. So one of the things we built into the James Cook University programme, to a lesser extent at Keele, and I've done it at other places since, was to expose students and immerse students in the much more positive environment of what works.

A comment about relationships: when I was a rural doc, it was probably the best network period of my life. I knew many peers who were similar to me. I had a network of urban specialists who would take a phone call from me 24 hours a day. If I really needed to talk to them I'd ring them once or twice a year at the most probably, and they knew that I would not abuse the privilege. But I actually think this contributed to, firstly, a very well supported rural workforce, those who did this, but secondly, I think it made for very good care. I find that the bigger the city I work in, the less accessible are all these people. You have to

---

[74] Hays (2003a).

refer people through fairly unknown channels, and they go on waiting lists, and they get triaged by people who wouldn't know anything about anything except following the triage algorithm. I'm not suggesting they don't do that well. I actually think that we've got this situation where rural practice can be extremely well networked. The threats to it are, funnily enough, technology. I think that a lot of doctors now, maybe all rural health professionals, believe that because they can go on the web – and where I come from, rural communities mostly have pretty good web access and bandwidth, but it's not universal – I think they talk to each other less and they seek help from these informal networks less and they rely on the same things that we've all got.

The second thing that is happening in terms of interprofessional stuff – I've also written about this. I think rural is almost the natural microcosm of interprofessional practice because everyone is so busy, they actually want to work together to share things and I think the outcomes are good.[75] But many of the health professions – I was interested in what Ivar was saying – while they have expanded their programmes to regional areas and some rural areas, it's actually harder to get rural allied health people now because no graduate, or very few graduates, from these programmes, feel confident enough to be generalists. In a sense, they are catching up with us in terms of moving out of urban settings but they haven't yet got the generalist/specialist balance to the point even we have in medicine. So I wonder if they might throw some interesting comments into the discussion.

Roger Strasser: Richard, you were at the beginning talking about the view a specialist and sub-specialist have and, you might say, the lens through which they were looking, it reminded me of rural proofing concepts that Jane mentioned and access to care for rural people.[76]

Randall-Smith: I would like to pick up on that but I wanted to link it back as well to the IT project that you were talking about because I think one of the most frustrating things is even when projects are successful, sometimes they're just not rolled out and made available. In the early/mid-1990s there were some really good telemedicine projects in mid-Wales and Shropshire but they disappeared.[77] The kit was taken out of the practices. Now we're talking about

---

[75] Hays (2007, 2008).

[76] See page 36.

[77] For example, in 1995, the Tele-Education and Medicine Project (TEAM) used video links to provide dermatology consultancy to rural GP practices in Powys, Wales. See Freeman *et al.* (1996).

major transformation programmes of how hospital services are delivered on the back of it, there are huge implications for general practice and community services but everybody's forgotten about the good work that was done 15–20 years ago. So they're almost reinventing the wheel again now. It just seems such a shame, especially when some of the education schemes, the dermatology, the consultant appointments, really, really benefited the patients and they liked them. You raise expectations and then it all disappears. Certainly locally they're talking about much more care delivered much closer to home and how they support the rural clinicians, maybe by GPs but there will also be advanced nurse practitioners and possibly physician assistants, but it feels like we're starting again. There's something about corporate memory there as well. Some of the things that are coming in are being dictated centrally and they've forgotten all about rural proofing, so what works in London or Birmingham isn't actually necessarily going to work in the more rural health economies. And because of times of austerity it's really focusing people's minds on how you deliver the services. There are huge opportunities for rural GPs but it's how you support them to actually deliver and be involved in the transformation. Even somewhere like Shropshire, which in the great scheme of things is not a huge area, you have to think about how different the practice is across the county. Although rural proofing was a really significant piece of work, it's very easy for people in positions of influence, because they've also got the funding, to forget about it because it suits them not to remember. And there just isn't that strength of opinion still. So it picks up on what John is saying. The rural voice is still not being heard and it's really, really frustrating. So I'm sorry, I don't know if I've taken the debate any further forward but I do think there are opportunities that we seem to forget very easily what we've learned.

Roger Strasser: We are learning about forgetting from the past, and also about history repeating itself. Hopefully this history being recorded will be learned from and not just blindly repeated.

Scott-Jones: I have a brief comment about the history of technology. I'm taking myself back to the end of this period of time that we're talking about, Y2K, when we all worried that the world was going to end with the change in the millennium.[78] And the thinking at the time, the thing that was helping us to network as rural GPs was teleconferencing, and Jim has also mentioned fax machines. What has struck me, although it does take us beyond 2000, is that

---

[78] Y2K (the year 2000) refers to a software problem at the turn of the millennium resulting from dates that had been stored in two-digit format, thus 1900 was indistinguishable from 2000.

basically we are, in New Zealand certainly, still reliant on very similar technology, and there are still issues in terms of our access to decent broadband. I have to say that this meeting is working incredibly well, compared to most of the experiences that I have with technology now. So times are changing. But during this period of time that we're talking about, it was basically telephones and teleconferences that linked us together and certainly we didn't have a significant network through social media or even a decent sort of email network of GPs working together.

The other thing I wanted to say was a little bit about education. During this period of time, certainly in New Zealand, we were picking up on a lot of what we were learning from Canada, and from Australia, in terms of getting people into rural communities out of the two main medical schools. It was during this time that longitudinal placements in practice were set up. There's been a change in landscape really in terms of how much general practice people get exposed to from the medical schools, which continues to this day. But what we saw was the establishment of these programmes during this time, and we've then seen a stagnation of things subsequently, in that there's a lack of will, incentive, or drive, to address the continued need for rural training. I think there's quite a bit about the urbanization of our country which is continuing. We now have 14 per cent of our population which is rural in the latest census, occupying 80 per cent of the land, but with no rural electorates. Although we have many politicians who have farming and rural backgrounds, there's not really a focus on the needs of rural communities, even though it's so central to our economy. Again, I think it's really interesting, thinking that it was 15 years ago that rural proofing was established in the UK – we're still struggling to try to get this implemented. Listening to the voices around the table reflecting on things I just feel like we are so far behind where the rest of the world is. Maybe I'm getting slightly depressed.

Račić: I think that technology is very important to family medicine in Bosnia because in many places we have surgeries where only one doctor works. So for them it's very important to have access to different conferences or seminars via technology like teleconferences. I can say that this probably in some part helps development of family medicine in Bosnia and Herzegovina. Jo said that 14 per cent of the whole population in New Zealand is rural, and I think it's much more in Bosnia.[79] So technology leads to very, very important issues. I

---

[79] According to the United Nations, Department of Economic and Social Affairs Population Division, 60.2 per cent of the population of Bosnia and Herzegovina was classed as living in rural areas in 2015; http://esa.un.org/unpd/wup/ (accessed 6 June 2016).

can also say that the health literacy of our patients improves with technology because, for example, when I started to work 20 years ago it was very different communicating with your patients than these days. I think it has significantly improved right now.

Wynn-Jones: Two areas I'd just like to mention. As you know, with John Togno we wrote the policy document on telemedicine and technology for the WONCA Working Party.[80] At the last meeting in Dubrovnik we acknowledged that that was out of date and should be reviewed. But if you actually look carefully, some of the comments we made are still highly relevant about technology possibly replacing well-trained physicians with local knowledge. I think that it's still relevant. The roll-out of technology has taken longer than we thought it would in rural areas. Looking back to the mid-1990s, when we set up the technology working group (WRITE) as part of the WONCA Working Party, there was a belief that telehealth was moving on faster. But things changed when the technicians and the politicians took over from the enthusiastic clinicians, and a bottom-up process was replaced by a top-down approach. Some of those telehealth innovations came from the bottom and were driven by the need to communicate over large distances. We took off-the-shelf technology and made it work, rather than using expensive forms of technology, which were purpose-built. So I have a little bit of scepticism about how it was rolled off and I agree with Jane. The paper is still relevant but it needs to be revised. Bandwidth is also a problem. It may not be a problem in some countries but in the mountainous areas of Wales and Scotland, it can be a problem and people are still without it. Interestingly, the chair of the rural forum of the RCGP still can't get proper internet access in Scotland.[81]

One more thing I'd just like to say about the urban/rural mix: I think we tend to think of rural as being agricultural and green, but there are pockets of industrialization, and now pockets of post-industrialization, that are clearly rural in every aspect in the sense that they're isolated. So we've got to be careful when we talk about occupational health, and occupational issues, and environmental issues in rural areas because, certainly in parts of Spain, you've got small coal mining communities that are now closing. We've seen this in the UK in parts of Wales and parts of England. So we've got to embrace those areas as well, and one of our great heroes, and one of my champions, Julian Hart, worked in

---

[80] WONCA (1998).

[81] Dr Malcolm Ward has chaired the RCGP Rural Forum since it was set up in 2009.

one of these isolated industrial communities.[82] I think Julian's very much a rural physician because many of the things we've talked about today, such as community involvement, about the health services being driven by the community, came from somebody who was seen as an urban advocate but was really rural. So it's how you define rurality, I think is going to be a difficult problem.

Rourke: Just touching on telemedicine and again focusing on technology, the 1970–2000 period was a very interesting time for telemedicine and, in fact, was led in the world by Dr Max House in Memorial – one of the first satellites to launch, the Anik B, had a Memorial medicine project on it.[83] Our geography really drove that because we had all these rural communities who were separated by either boat or airplane flights, served by nurses; what the telemedicine allowed them to do was connect up to the rural doctors who could support them and allow the patients to stay in those rural communities with the proper support network. Then where that developed, further along that line, avoids all sorts of transfers from rural communities to larger centres because we've got specialists who will support the rural doctors in telemedicine, all developing over that time period. Around the world telemedicine came in and money was spent on pilot projects and they disappeared when the money ran out. But in our setting it was found to be extremely cost-effective so it has become built into the healthcare system just like the telephone – it's ubiquitous. We don't even think about it anymore, it's just such a part of our routine practice, and it allows the patients to stay in their own communities instead of coming in for cancer follow-up, or visitor psychiatry consults, in the tertiary care centres at a huge cost to the patient and disruption to the family. Those things can all be done by telemedicine and really it's one of the things that has stayed now the technology's changed, but it really has allowed for improvement of access in our particular context instead of reduction of access as has happened in other areas. And it's been a sustainable thing because it's looked at for cost-effectiveness and it's been very cost-effective.

---

[82] Dr Julian Tudor Hart (b. 1927) was a GP in South Wales from 1961 to 1988; from 1968 he conducted independent epidemiological research. He contributed to the Witness Seminars on 'Population-based Research in South Wales': Ness, Reynolds, and Tansey (eds) (2002) and 'Research in general practice': Reynolds and Tansey (eds) (1998). An interview with Dr Tudor Hart is available on our website at www. histmodbiomed.org/

[83] Dr (Arthur) Maxwell House (1926–2013) was Professor of Neurology at Memorial University of Newfoundland, Canada, and from 1997 to 2002 was Lieutenant-Governor of Newfoundland and Labrador. In 1976 he founded the Telemedicine Centre and the telehealth programme at Memorial. See Scott (2013). For the early years of telemedicine at Memorial see, for example, Elford (2009), and for the use of satellites see Chouinard (1983).

I wanted to segue in from there to something we haven't talked about and I think we'll get to, and that's the sustainability of rural practice. We tend to focus so much on educating doctors for rural practice, but at the end of the day if the work is not something that's well supported by the community, by the healthcare system, by the networks in place, by the funding incentives, then creating this big pipeline to rural practice and have it land on the rocks of rural practice that are going to be unforgiving or unsupportive, it won't really get us where we need.[84] We've seen some places, like in Australia and some parts of Canada, where rural practice becomes much more supported and is made more attractive and sustainable, but other areas that have fallen way behind and are not places where people would or could work for a long time. I just wonder whether that's maybe an area that people have got a lot of comments on, as well as about that aspect of how you make the workplace something that's going to be a place that's going to attract graduates with all their educational effort that has been put into it.

Douglas: I just really want to come back to the point of social accountability and equity. Let's get off the technology because I think we've done technology to death, and really come back to the period that we're talking about, 1970–2000, and develop the theme that Bruce Chater was talking about, about how young doctors, young GPs, are saying you shouldn't be close to your patients.[85] I think certainly if we're thinking in an historical sense of what happened between the period of 1970–2000, a generation of doctors sitting around this room, like Bruce Chater who sat in his rural community for 35 years, like me who sat in my rural community for 35 years, like John Wynn-Jones who sat in his rural community for similar sorts of time – we're a generation that have been about commitment and we probably reflect really the social norms of the day. So during this time period I think relationships, marriage, and so on, were for long periods of time. I'm still married to my wife after 37 years – how she puts up with me I don't know. But relationships were long term. We're now into a society where we have a sort of serial monogamy, where relationships are maybe shorter and I think certainly one of the defining things about that time period of 1970–2000 was this sense of commitment to a community and a sense of responsibility to that community. If I just take it down to my own level and what happened to me: I felt, sitting in my community, I observed things round about to make sure that history didn't repeat itself. So, for instance, when I went in as a young doctor to my community, I saw occupational health problems

---

[84] See, for example, Rourke *et al.* (2003).

[85] See page 60.

related to the aluminium factory and people with dreadful COPD (chronic obstructive pulmonary disease). That was a driver therefore for when another industry came into the area – fish processing – I didn't want to see history repeating itself.[86] The driver came for me at a personal level, it was of a long-term commitment to this community and not wanting to see damage done again to that community. Another example would be that somebody was talking about organophosphate pesticides. Well, when I started in my community I spent my time worrying about organophosphate pesticides being used by sheep farmers and getting long-term neurological-effects, and a lot of campaigning and so on about that. Now, 35 years later, I'm worrying about Lyme neuroborreliosis because of lack of sheep. The environment has changed – we don't have sheep going around cleaning up the bracken and getting rid of the ticks, the sheep are not dipped by organophosphate pesticides, the cycle has continued. So I'm now spending my time worrying about the neurological impacts of people who work on the land but it's not the pesticides this time, it's now the ticks. So there's something about this time period we're looking at, about commitment, about being in it for the long term, about being the clinical scientist, being the observer, etc. And I think things are changing. I certainly can relate to what Bruce Chater is saying. I'm a little bit horrified by some of the things that I'm hearing from some of the young doctors, and obviously medicine has to reflect the society that it serves but definitely cultural values are changing. I suppose my final point is, if we are looking back on this period, somebody is reading this report in 50 years' time, we have had, during this period that we're talking about, a particular set of cultural norms and sets of cultural values and social accountability, and that's the observation that I wish to make.

Rourke: It's a calling, not an opportunity.

Sarah Strasser: What I've been thinking about as we've been discussing, is that at the WONCA Crete conference, Barbara Starfield challenged us to define the role of the specialist.[87] Not that I want to go back to that particular argument, but I think it fits in with this business about proper support networks and specialists acting as true consultants to the rural physician, and in fact the rural physician

---

[86] See page 34.

[87] Professor Barbara Starfield (1932—2011) was University Distinguished Service Professor and Professor of Health Policy and Pediatrics at Johns Hopkins University. She gave the keynote speech 'The contribution of primary care to equity: How and what do we do now?' at the ninth WONCA Rural Health Conference, held in Heraklion, Crete, in June 2009. The PowerPoint slides from this speech have been archived with the records of this meeting in Archives and Manuscripts, Wellcome Library, London, at GC/253.

to the mid-level worker. My concern is that, as Barbara Starfield and others have pointed out, that the costs of care are increasing way beyond any improvement in care that is happening. I think that we have a need to work out this business of the mid-level care workers and how we support them and determine how the specialists support us because all the things that are coming into the hospitals at the moment in the big cities are about reducing costs. This is just shifting the load back to general practice and the community. I have a fear that the cost implications are such that it will be mid-level care workers who are cut out. It will be the generalists, and particularly the care in the community, that will be cut out unless we have your system, Jim, of being able to declare that things like telemedicine are cost-effective. So we really have to home in on those because I don't think the average politician or bureaucrat is seeing that the highest cost is the sheer abundance of administrators and the sub-specialists who've all got their own little special areas of interest so that they will no longer go beyond their own interests, who have become part of the healthcare system. It's going to have a negative impact if we don't pick up the issues that are beneficial yet are getting lost, which we've learned from experience and are talking about in this Witness Seminar.

Roger Strasser: I think you've set the stage really for our last round of discussion as we complete this because we are committed to finish this seminar within the timeframe that was set. So it's not a long-term commitment in that sense. Sarah mentioned Barbara Starfield, and just to enlarge on her contribution really to the knowledge of healthcare, which was to demonstrate, through studies in looking at almost every country in the world, every part of the world, and many different health systems, that the most efficient and effective, cost-effective health services, is comprehensive primary healthcare.[88] So where we have a comprehensive primary healthcare as part of the health system, then the health outcomes are better and the costs are lower. That was when she said: 'Well, that's what you do, rural doctors, that's what you provide. So what do the specialists do?' And that was the challenge that she gave to us, and, as Sarah's just said now, one of the challenges for us is actually countering the bean-counters who are always looking at unit cost. You need to look at the big picture, look at the overall return on investment. Government, other organizations, tend to be departmentalized and they just look at their own budget, their own cost, and ignore other costs and often quite comfortably offload those costs.

---

[88] See, for example, Starfield, Shi, and Macinko (2005).

I do want to bring this discussion to an end, so we're now including those sort of final themes. Social accountability and equity has been mentioned. The WONCA had a role with the World Health Organization in 1994; there was a conference in London, Ontario, which was focused on producing doctors responding to community need.[89] The next year, 1995, the World Health Organization produced a formal definition of the social accountability of medical schools,[90] and that movement was gaining momentum in the latter 1990s and has been taken further into the 2000s. Gender, we've heard about the increasing number of women in medicine; I think it's fair to say that up until the 1970s and maybe a bit later in some countries, that the characteristic rural doctor was a bullet-proof super doc, could do everything – that was rather a male macho kind of image. A question then is the wife, and where does the wife fit in, and the family? So some points maybe for discussion there. So we've described rural doctors living in the community they serve – for the family it's like living in a fishbowl, with people always watching and commenting what they do, and those sort of dimensions. The sustainability issue has already been raised – certainly the themes mentioned about education and training, financial, personal, and professional supports – I think that one that's often not given the attention it needs is models of healthcare delivery that are sustainable. John Wynn-Jones made the comment about maintaining surgical and maternity services, and there's been some research in British Columbia that connects the two,[91] and really if you lose one you lose the other, and then there's a downward spiral in terms of the capacity of the local hospital and healthcare providers. So that's setting the scene for our final round.

What I'm going to do is strictly alphabetically because I want to give everyone a chance to make a final comment, but you only have a minute each. So this requires some discipline and I know it's more of a challenge for some than others. [Laughter] Who was it that said: 'I don't have time to be brief?' I'm going to start, alphabetical first around the virtual table and then around the physical table here in London. So we'll start with Ivar Aaraas. Your final comment – you have one minute, Ivar.

Aaraas: My final comment is about the relationship between rural and specialist healthcare. During the period 1970–2000 the impact of specialization, including building of large hospitals, was very strong. In Norway, before 1970, we had a lot

---

[89] A joint World Health Organization and WONCA conference was held in Ontario, Canada in November 1994: World Health Organization/WONCA (1995).

[90] Boelen and Heck (1995).

[91] See, for example, Humber and Frecker (2008).

of rural community hospitals run by GPs (also called cottage hospitals), which were closed down. Now we have a strong counter-force to rebuild this kind of small rural hospital, and that has to do with many things. One thing is about technology (tele-technology), another about modern transportation, which makes transfer of patients easier and travel time shorter. The easier transportation of patients to and from the big hospitals, including use of tele-technology, gives the small hospitals a much more profound role. They can observe patients before they are sent, or often don't send them because they can cope with the situation locally, sometimes with tele-technological support from a large hospital. And the rural hospital can safely take back patients earlier, as time in the busy large hospitals is getting increasingly shorter. I think this situation is favourable for renewing the role of the small rural hospitals in the future.[92]

Chater: I'd just like to make a couple of comments. I think this time in the late 1990s/early 2000s, one of the saddest things was seeing the loss of many mentors and facilities – I think what Ivar was just saying about rural hospitals being closed. We're starting to catch up a little bit in Australia about getting the data about the cost-efficiencies of those hospitals – I've talked to many of you about some of the data that we've managed to get in Australia recently about the cost-efficiency. I think we can build on that with technology. We're just about to look at tele-chemotherapy back in our rural hospitals; we're now doing tele-pharmacy in our rural hospitals. So we're using the technology to re-establish things, but I think the late 1990s/early 2000s were probably starting to be a little bit of a low point with the facilities that we had. I think trying to turn that around has been a significant challenge because of the loss of, as I said, mentors and facilities.

Couper: I want to just reflect back, and it's interesting, I know Bruce is not negative generally, but his comments were maybe a bit negative, and I want to take the positive slant. If we look back at where we have come from, there have been some very positive developments and forward movements over the years. I think Richard, to some extent, reflected on that in terms of how education has changed, that when we talk about rural health education people don't raise their eyebrows and kind of think we're mad. It's now an accepted part of education in many parts of the world. We have departments, or centres, or chairs of rural health and rural practice, etc. That's become normative and that's important in terms of the development of training and changing the way training is happening. I think the WHO, recognizing that rural has an important place with the 2010 guidelines

---

[92] Aaraas *et al.* (2000).

that were produced[93] and the more recent *Transforming Health Professions Education*,[94] again has been mainstreaming some of those issues internationally. It's not to say we don't still face many challenges in trying to make the difference and that notion that, Roger, you referred to earlier about the solution some people think is for everybody just to be urbanized and then we've dealt with the problem. That thinking is unfortunately still there in many people, but I think there is an increasing recognition that no one can get away from having to address the rural issue ultimately in one way or another, whether they want to or not. I think that's been a significant development. Linking back also to the earlier discussion around specialists: in my early days specialist outreach was quite common, it's now coming back as something that actually all specialists must know about, outreach and the health system, coming to models of healthcare, must be a system that is reaching out rather than people having to reach out to the system.

Hamilton: I just return but in this context to something I talked about before. Be you rural or be you urban, you will have disadvantaged groups for some similar and some different reasons. And unless we study the community on its own terms we will not fully understand the scope or the remedies for that. So I think in education, postgraduate education, and selection of students, you need to be exploring and representing those problems. When we have Aboriginal students coming into the class, the whole class changed its point of view about Aboriginal welfare. I've had five students lately working with the prison rescue group, that is a group of volunteers who get youngsters coming out of prison and help them get back into society. They are teaching our medical students and half of them are ex-cons. They've been in prison themselves, they've known what it's like and they can teach people to spot the risk factors, know how to rescue them, and all that. That's investment for the future for cost, all sorts of things. So the real world is where I think the medical schools need to be. You've heard me say that many times. [Laughs]

Roger Strasser: But we're in the real world and we're talking about the real, rural world.

Hamilton: But urban world or rural world, you still have to take the same approach to get out into the community and learn on their terms. It's a false dichotomy to say that there's a totally different approach. You need a common ground of approach and learn from each other.

---

[93] World Health Organization (2010).

[94] World Health Organization (2013).

Inem: Essentially I want to say that between 1970 and now, we in the rural areas have not concentrated much on gender issues, especially in terms of violence to women in rural areas. We are trying now to put this into the curriculum for rural residents so that they can have skills to take care of some of these issues. That takes me also to the issue of the less privileged, like you have mentioned the prisoners and so on, who are in society. In fact, some of our prisons are more or less in the rural areas and we are getting to learn quite a lot from them. It's just that our Government has not been too forthcoming in encouraging the interaction between the family physician and the services. Presently we have an ongoing issue of IDPs (internally displaced persons) in the north-east of the country, and even though we have skilled manpower to be there, not much is being done, except for what we had done earlier on in the south-west of the country when Liberia, Sierra Leone, and some of these other countries, were using Nigeria as a transit point when there were refugees. We took them right into the rural areas and we thought, for example, we had a problem of their bringing in infectious diseases into Nigeria in which we compared the HIV (human immunodeficiency virus) rates of the refugees with those of the indigenous and found out that in fact there was no difference. Even though there was that fear that these people were going to bring in new infections, new infestations, into the community, that was not our experience. So rural areas can be quite safe and can be used as a veritable training ground for most of our doctors both at undergraduate and postgraduate levels.

Kravtchenko: Just a short comment regarding emerging technologies. I believe we shouldn't underestimate it and it's not only the use of social media but it's also communication use, such as communication between doctor and patient, doctor and other medical professionals, and communication between doctors. And not only use of wire technology such as the internet but also wireless, mobile phones, and the usage is increasing and it's been increased tremendously since 1970, if we look back. I guess perhaps it's time to prepare some projects to improve and perhaps go ahead of information technology companies such as Intel and Apple. I know that some programmes like this already exist, and it's point of care ECG and ultrasound, and all these other techniques which save time initially, and they could be used in the education of young physicians and give increasing access to healthcare in rural areas. I believe expectations of people in rural areas are increasing and are being increased dramatically. So I guess, perhaps this IT gives not only a challenge but also a tremendous opportunity to further develop healthcare.

Pekez-Pavlisko: I think in the past century we had two ways, two organizations of rural medicine: in some parts like Canada, Australia, South Africa, United States; in south-east Europe and some parts of African and Asia actually rural medicine decreased a lot and I think it's time that we re-establish our power and our leadership and management in all parts of the world. That's it from me, very short.

Račić: I just wanted to comment that John Hamilton made a really good point because sometimes, and I notice during conversation, urban doctors often have prejudice towards rural doctors and rural medicine. But it seems to me that we are starting to behave similarly, so we really need to find a common approach in order to improve undergraduate education, postgraduate education, and actually the ultimate goal will be to have better healthcare in one country. I think we really need to show to our colleagues the good examples, what changes will be made if we include rural doctors and rural hospitals into the teaching process.

Randall-Smith: I too would like to pick up what John Hamilton said about understanding the needs of people and of communities; I think that's really, really important. I'd also like to address the other level that I don't think locally, or across Europe, rural practice still has the recognition that it deserves, so I think it's very important we try to get that rural voice heard, that rural practice might be different. So it comes back to rural proofing, which then links back to listening to that local voice and meeting those local needs.

Scott-Jones: I consider myself a Thatcher refugee and left the UK during that period of time. I think the centralization of services began at that time and actually you talked about social accountability; I think there was a sense of reduction of social accountability in terms of particularly rural community services because of that focus on the economic efficiency of the services and of the communities. And we still see that centralization of the provision of services rolling on. I think also during this period of time, for us in New Zealand, there was a reduction of engagement of spouses in our rural general practice network. We'd modelled ourselves on the Australian Family Network and we saw a reduction of that. I wondered if that was a reflection of the societal change that has been raised earlier on – change in attitude towards autonomy and a focus on the importance of individuals as opposed to collective responsibility that we saw during that time. Again, I think we're still seeing that having ongoing impact. I think it was also a time when we saw the beginning of the feminization of the workforce of medicine. We know we now have the majority of medical graduates being female, which has yet to have impact on our rural workforce, but we haven't really touched on that change, an important change in gender identity of our medical workforce. But, again, during this time in New Zealand it was the energy of rural champions like Pat Farry and Tim Malloy,[95] who were supported by their international connections and they are known to people around the table, and that was their energy supported by you, the international connections they had, and international evidence that provided a platform for developing undergraduate education in New Zealand at that time. What we've seen subsequently is a focus more on postgraduate rural education in New Zealand.

Wynn-Jones: Just a few comments. I agree with Ian Couper; I think we mustn't forget the huge advances that happened. You know when we first started, rural wasn't on the agenda in the UK, it wasn't on the agenda in Europe, and I think we've worked hard to try and develop that and so I think there has been a move forward. I would also just like to reiterate some of John Hamilton's words that he said. Rural and urban areas do have similar problems, just the context is different. I always work on the principle that, if it works in rural, it will work in urban because I think the constraints are often going to be greater in rural. That's the first thing I would say. I think the other thing, as far as good news and bad news, was that towards the end of that period of 1970–2000 I would see as the golden age of general practice in the UK. Some people were diametrically opposed to the concept of fund-holding but, in fact, it worked well and it certainly worked well in our rural area. We were empowered, we had teams working together, there was a bottom-up approach, and I think it's very, very sad.[96] So I suppose I'm thinking ahead and thinking of the next seminar. Most of us probably won't be here for that but it'll be looking back on the years 2000–2030. I think we'll be saying how all these issues are cyclical – we've seen the cyclical changes that have occurred and it'll happen again.

---

[95] Dr Patrick Farry (1944–2009) was a GP in Queenstown, New Zealand, and was Medical Director of Te Waipounamu Rural Health Unit at the Dunedin School of Medicine where he had responsibility for undergraduate and postgraduate studies in Rural Health. He established the Rural Medical Immersion Programme (RMIP) in 2007. Dr Tim Malloy was chair of the Rural General Practitioners' Chapter of the Royal New Zealand College of General Practitioners, and has been President of the College since 2012.

[96] General Practice fund-holding, whereby practices could hold and manage their budget, was introduced by the Conservative Government in 1991. The scheme was abolished by the Labour Government in 1998; see, for example, Dixon and Glennerster (1995); and for its abolition, Kay (2002).

Just some of the sad things that have happened: I agree with Bruce entirely. I think we've had a loss of empathy and I sent around something to the Google group about the Empathy Museum and I think, sadly, it is a museum because in fact we've lost some of that.[97] Austerity is beginning to have a worsening impact in Europe and I think it's having an impact around the world. We've also seen in the period of time, 1970–2000, horrendous times in Europe and horrendous times in other parts of the world. To think that there were wars in the Balkans and that's had an impact on rural health. And we're swapping the impact of war now for the impact of migration, and that's going to be a big change and it's going to have a huge impact on European health and on European rural health. So a mixed feeling, some really good news, some great things happened in that period of time but you can see the portent of worrying things to come. So you'd better start appointing whoever is going to take over from you, Roger, for the next time round in the next 30 years. So thanks a lot.

Roger Strasser: Well, I don't know about me actually but I was thinking actually, so if it's 2030, it'll be 15 years later, 2045, will you be up for it, Tilli?

Tansey: I don't think so! Most of us will be very, very elderly if we're still here. [Laughter]

Roger Strasser: Don't think so? Okay, well, it's Tilli that needs to find someone.

Sarah Strasser: Some very wise words from a dear colleague of ours who has since died, Robert Hall, were that the rural decline has been happening for hundreds of years and it's not going to go away.[98] So basically we need to get on and do something about it. I think what John Wynn-Jones was just hinting at in business terms is called 'reverse innovation'. They are truly finding that you can't just adapt a business model and plonk it in a rural or developing country and expect it to work. You actually have to go with an open mind, create something that actually solves the problem, without the constraints of the urban or developed country mindset, and then you will get the real thing. We can't afford to forget that this can then become a world winner and that we can actually lead the field. So I think that's a positive note and that's where I'm going to end.

---

[97] The Empathy Museum was set up in 2015 to explore, through events and installation, 'how empathy can not only transform our personal relationships but also help tackle global challenges such as prejudice, conflict and inequality'; see www.empathymuseum.com/ (accessed 13 April 2016).

[98] Dr Robert Hall (d. 2014) worked as a rural GP in Gippsland, Victoria, and was an educator and a founder member of the Monash University Centre for Rural Health. See Professor Roger Strasser's tribute, 'Farewell Robert Hall – Truly One of a Kind', on the WONCA website at: www.globalfamilydoctor.com/News/FarewellRobertHallTrulyOneofaKind.aspx (accessed 1 June 2016).

Douglas: I would like to end this seminar on the topic of history and the importance of historical discourse on rural practice because I think history, and the analysis of history, is a very useful method that we've recently been using in Scotland to advance the political process and to engage with change. As everybody knows we've got a long history in the UK of medical education, going back 500 years or so, and our history in terms of rural practice goes back about 100 years. The world's first report on remote and rural general practice was done in 1912, the Dewar Report in the Highlands and Islands of Scotland.[99] The important thing about that report is it then led on to being the rural challenges that were described at that time then led on to the establishment of the National Health Service in 1948, which has really defined our healthcare during the period that we're looking at today between 1970 and 2000. More recently, in 2012, I was part of the historical collaboration that looked at that history again for a new generation to refresh it, and to use it to engage with politicians. The historical point is that we were able to say there was a problem, it was described in this document in 1912, this is what they did about it, and this is what is happening now. We are able to use that process as a very neutral document where we're able to reflect back and say: 'These are the problems in 2012, this is what you need to do about it', because part of the difficulty we have in the UK is political involvement within the health service.[100]

So I think history and historical discourse is really important and I would like to end finally by saying we now have a new icon of rural general practice. About 100 years ago, there was a guy called Lachlan Grant from Ballachulish – his biography was published two weeks ago and is an absolutely fascinating life-history of a rural doctor. He came from that community, he went away to university, he came back to serve that community throughout his whole life.[101] He engaged with national level politicians, he was a good clinical scientist, and he was a good social reformer and good clinician. So there are many things where historical discourse can teach us lessons for today. I'd like to finally thank Tilli and Roger for engaging with this historical discourse because it's really important.

---

[99] Highlands and Islands Medical Service Committee Report (1912) Cmd 6559 (Dewar Report), available online at www.elib.scot.nhs.uk/Upload/Dewar_Report.pdf (accessed 13 April 2016). For a fuller discussion of the Dewar Report, see pages 87–8.

[100] The Dewar 2012 Group was set up to commemorate the 100th anniversary of the Dewar Report. See the website of the group at http://ruralgp.com/dewar2012/ (accessed 1 June 2016).

[101] Dr Lachlan Grant (1871–1945) was a GP and scientist in the Western Highlands of Scotland. He was an active campaigner for economic and social reform, was involved in industrial disputes, and was a leading contributor to the Dewar Report of 1912. Cameron and Tindley (2015).

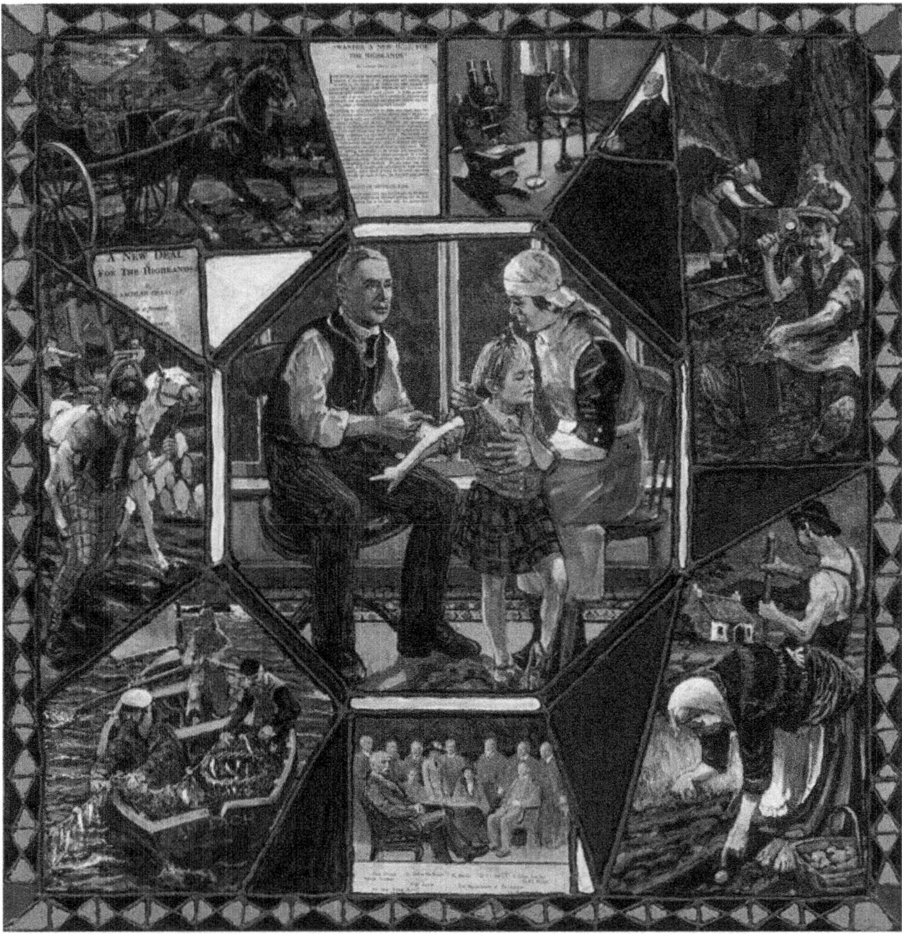

Figure 27: Painting celebrating Dr Lachlan Grant's contribution to rural health.
Artist: Mr Alastair Smyth, DA, commissioned by Dr James Douglas and
presented to the Royal College of General Practitioners, Edinburgh[102]

Rourke: Well, thank you, and I'll start off on my thanks to Tilli and Roger. I think this is an important discourse so thank you for doing this and it's such a pleasure to be here with the people who have contributed so much to this time period of 1970–2000. When I look back on that I think one of the most

---

[102] 'The central pane shows Grant immunizing a child; the pony and trap are a reference to transport problems for doctors in the Highlands and Islands; the laboratory pane refers to his active research career; the Highland crofters, fishermen and forestry workers were his patients; the slate quarry workers were his occupational health interest. The Dewar Committee in the bottom sepia pane were the official conduit for his vision for a NHS and Ramsay MacDonald M.P. and Prime Minister in the top small triangle, became his friend and correspondent.' Douglas, Tindley, and Smyth (2015), page 234.

significant things is the development of a professional identity for rural doctors at that time, developed by people for whom rural practice was truly a calling. I'm thinking of Dr MacLeod, Dr M K Rajakumar, other people, and the people around our teleconference today.[103] I'm privileged to be part of that group. It developed a positive profile for rural physicians, which I think has been significant in helping move some things forward. One of them is developing strong rural education programmes and the move in many areas to produce better supports for rural doctors and rural practitioners and rural healthcare in rural communities. But the goal of health for our rural people, which was one of our initiatives, is not an eight-lane superhighway, it's a wandering road through the bush with many unexpected challenges along the way, or a stormy ocean passage with cliffs and reefs that you have to avoid. Rural practice still faces those challenges, but we have a whole cadre of people now involved in rural practice as rural doctors, and hopefully we'll take this forward because I do think it is a need that still requires high-profile leadership to maintain the focus on providing health to the people in communities, which is what people around here have been working on all this time. So an exciting time period but it will remain a challenge, as Robert Hall, said, forever; and if we let up on it we will lose the challenge.[104]

Roger Strasser: The price of liberty is eternal vigilance.

Hays: So adversity drives innovation. We were part of a group, many of us who came out of the 1970s and 1980s and 1990s, in Australia; the problems were well known, they'd been identified, written in endless reports, and a bunch of people, only a small proportion of whom we've heard mentioned, really drove change and got things done. I think I'd want to look forward. In terms of sustainability we need to think about how this is going to keep going. I'm now in Tasmania trying to re-ruralize a healthcare system facing immense challenges because the hospitals are closed and most of the health professionals, apart from medicine, have been deskilled with a narrower scope of practice. The workforce in medicine is now much more female, it's younger, and there are people who are not going to stay there for 35 years. I believe we need to engage these people in finding the solutions to the current set of challenges which will take us forward – I'm the eternal optimist; I think they're there.

---

[103] For Dr John MacLeod, see page 35 and note 40, and comments on page 106–7; and for Dr M K Rajakumar, see page 59 and note 73.

[104] See page 76.

Roger Strasser: Well, thank you, Richard, and potentially taking up the reverse innovation approach that Sarah mentioned, I think that we, certainly in the rural movement, have been challenging the conventional wisdom that says anything that happens outside the big cities is second class, and in fact there's a lot that the cities or the urban areas can learn from rural. But agreeing certainly with John Hamilton the importance of context and it's the realities of communities wherever they are. I think there are specific dimensions to the rural context and certainly a key issue is that access is the rural health issue. Even in countries where most of the people live in rural areas, the resources are concentrated in the cities, there are always transport and communication difficulties from one rural area to another, and between the rural and the urban settings, and there continue to be shortages of doctors and other health professionals in those rural areas. So reflecting on rural practice, rural medicine, during that time period, the 1970s to 2000, and I think we've heard, it's fair to say, that rural medicine did develop, become recognized and accepted as a distinct discipline and with the specific characteristics that rural practitioners are members of the community that they serve and they focus on responding to the needs of the community. It's that sense of being part of a community and responding to community needs, and that rural practitioners, when compared to their metropolitan counterparts, are extended generalists. They provide a wider range of services and carry a higher level of clinical responsibility in relative professional isolation, and as they are members of the community that they serve they influence the health of the community, the whole community, a population health sort of approach. Back to access: a key role of the rural practitioner is access to primary, secondary, and tertiary care, whether it's having the skills and the support to provide secondary care locally or ensuring that the patients have secondary care and the tertiary care in whatever system that you're working.

We've covered a lot of ground together over the last almost four hours – I've certainly thoroughly enjoyed this. I want to thank all of you for your participation, particularly those of you who have managed to stay awake through the night, especially in New Zealand and Australia. From my point of view it was absolutely worth it and I do want to say thank you very much to the team here, who have brought this together. To Caroline and to Adam, who you all met by email and now those with video have seen, and to Professor Tilli Tansey for initiating this Witness Seminar, and we're certainly looking forward to the record and the opportunity to share this when it is published. I think Tilli wants to make some closing remarks.

Tansey: Yes, I'm going to add my thanks. This has been a great afternoon for those of us who have not participated but have listened to your reminiscences and reflections. Clearly this period was one of considerable change in social relations, in technology, general culture and professional training, practice, and expectations. What's come out quite clearly is not only the change but the commonalities as some of you have reached out to each other across national boundaries, and the importance of the creation of national and international organizations really struck me. One thing that does surprise me is how little this area is examined by professional historians of medicine. This is something I'd certainly like to address in the future. I'd like to add my thanks to those of Roger's to all of you who have participated, particularly our three colleagues for whom this is the middle of the night. I have to say I was very impressed that none of you logged in wearing your pyjamas, which is what I'd slightly expected.

Roger Strasser: Look – Jo is wearing his pyjamas. [Laughter, as Jo Scott-Jones removes his jumper to reveal pyjamas]

Tansey: I'm particularly grateful to Roger – I'm sure you all are – for his excellent chairing, summing up, his getting us all around in time, and thank you to the Wellcome Trust for the technology.

THE HISTORY OF RURAL MEDICINE AND RURAL MEDICAL EDUCATION

The transcript of a Witness Seminar held by the
Wellcome Trust Centre for the History of Medicine
at UCL, on 29 January 2010

THE HISTORY OF RURAL MEDICINE AND RURAL MEDICAL EDUCATION

Participants*

Dr Gordon Baird
Dr Jim Cox
Dr James Douglas
Professor Richard Hays
Dr David Hogg
Dr Iain McNicol

Professor Sir Eldryd Parry
Professor Sir Denis Pereira Gray (Chair)
Professor Roger Strasser
Professor Sarah Strasser
Professor Tilli Tansey

* Biographical notes on the participants are located at the end of the volume

Professor Tilli Tansey: Thank you all very much for coming to this Witness Seminar on the 'History of Rural Medicine and Rural Medical Education'. One of the things this programme in the history of contemporary biomedicine tries to do is create synergies between practitioners and historians, and we've devised this format of the Witness Seminar. We invite a number of people from a range of backgrounds to meet together and join in open and frank discussion. The suggestion of a Witness Seminar in rural medicine came from John Hamilton in Australia and Roger Strasser in Canada. Several efforts to set up a meeting of rural medicine of our usual size, of 20 to 25 participants, have been unsuccessful because of conflicting appointments, etc. Recently, however, my colleague Lois Reynolds and I have run, with the Wellcome Trust Policy Unit, some smaller Witness Seminars.[105] These have each had 10–12 people, and they've been so extremely successful that we decided to adopt a similar format for rural medicine. We have in front of us an agenda with a rough outline of topics we think might

<table>
<tr><td>

Practice: provision and maintenance of services
- Rural Medicine/RARM (Remote and Rural Medicine): when did it start? Who did it, where, why, and how?
- Isolated practitioners as service providers: problems and potentials; what level of service provision?
- Teamwork: the history of all the players?
- National and international organizations: how did they start and why? Networks and communications

Education
- Needs of students bound for rural practice
- National
- International (training for the colonies?)
- Academic developments
- Role of professional organizations

The future of the history of RARM
- How to record it? How to study it? Who to do it?
- Future connections?

</td></tr>
</table>

Table 2: Outline programme for the Witness Seminar
'The History of Rural Medicine and Rural Medical Education'

---

[105] Professor Tilli Tansey and Mrs Lois Reynolds contributed to the Wellcome Trust Portfolio Reviews: *Human Genetics 1990–2009* (2010), https://wellcome.ac.uk/sites/default/files/wtx063661_0.pdf; *Human Functional Brain Imaging 1990–2009* (2011), https://wellcome.ac.uk/sites/default/files/wtvm052606.pdf; and *Malaria 1990–2009* (2012), https://wellcome.ac.uk/sites/default/files/wtvm054952_0.pdf (all accessed 6 February 2017).

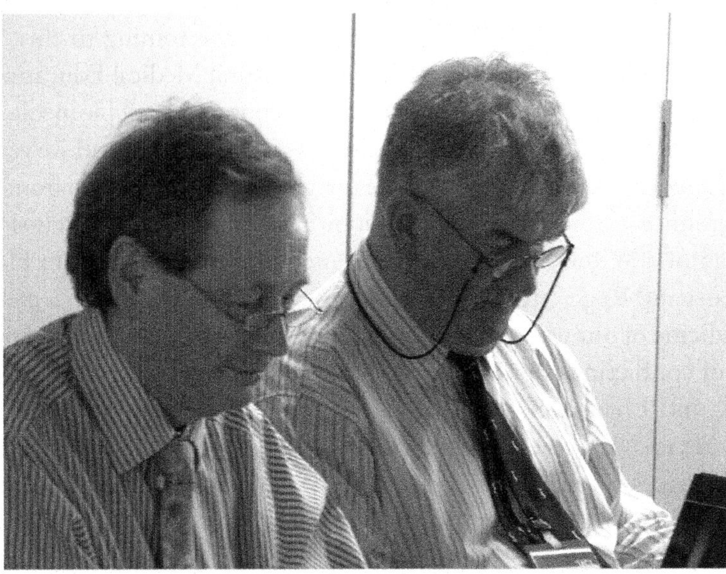

Figure 28: Dr James Douglas and Dr Iain McNicol

be important to discuss (Table 2), but if there are topics that we've missed out that you would like to raise please do so, this is your meeting. An important part of any meeting is identifying a suitable chairman, and I was delighted that Sir Denis Pereira Gray agreed to chair this meeting to keep you all in order.

Professor Sir Denis Pereira Gray: Thank you very much, Tilli. I think we're all very grateful to the Wellcome Trust and Tilli and her team here for setting this up. The Witness Seminars are a great tradition and this size is a very attractive group to give everybody a chance to speak and discuss and think about the topics we have been working on. Let me say at the beginning that I'm not an expert on rural medicine, I spent my life as an urban general practitioner but I have a very great interest in the subject and have a lot of colleagues and friends in rural practice. I think it's a particular pleasure today that we've got international visitors – from Canada and Australia – they are particularly welcome; they will be taking a broad perspective on this subject. If we look at the agenda, you will see it's been divided up into a service part and then an educational part. The heading we've got for the first part is 'Practice: provision and maintenance of services', which is broad enough to give us all a chance to get going. So the floor is open.

Dr James Douglas: Although this is the history of rural medicine in the twentieth century I think it would be useful to focus on what we know about the history of rural medicine in the UK and the question about where it all started. I'm actually an NHS general practitioner in Fort William on the west coast of Scotland. I've been there 30 years and Fort William is a rural town with a wide hinterland. I've had an interest in rural medicine and rural health throughout those 30 years and my two areas of particular interest are education and operational health.

If we look at the history, we have a history of ancient universities in the UK – the University of Aberdeen was started in 1495 and claims to have the first chair of medicine in the UK, but really if we come on to the first definitions of what is remote and rural healthcare and what are the problems, the first documentary evidence that we have is undoubtedly what the university referred to as the Dewar Report of 1912, the investigation by the Highlands and Islands Medical Committee.[106] That's interesting because there are many lessons from that report, which are still relevant today, and some of the themes that Dewar drew out about education, about service delivery, about generalism, and so on are as true today in many ways as they were in 1912. An interesting thing about the Dewar Report is that it all started because of the lack of data going to Government. Government was desperate to get information, it wasn't being properly filled in. In Skye, despite the fact that there were doctors there and the Government of the day decided that although there were doctors in the remote and rural parts of Scotland some of them were good at filling in the death certificates but some of them were obviously pretty poor. So a very big committee of the Government, a committee of inquiry, went round the whole of Scotland, around the Highlands and Islands, in a systematic qualitative methodology – we would call it qualitative methodology now – and drew out themes. The basic facts were that the poor people couldn't pay the attendance fees of the doctors and the doctors were very variable. They fell into two categories of rural doctor: there was the person with missionary zeal and missionary accomplishments and then there was the drunkard who was absolutely useless. What this committee of

---

[106] Highlands and Islands Medical Service Committee Report (1912) Cmd 6559 (Dewar Report), available online at www.elib.scot.nhs.uk/Upload/Dewar_Report.pdf (accessed 13 April 2016). Sir John Dewar (1856–1929) was MP for Inverness-shire from 1900 to 1916. For the Dewar centenary see comments by Dr James Douglas at the 2015 Witness Seminar on page 77. Professor Sir Denis Pereira Gray wrote: 'It was a good report and very influential for rural medicine in Scotland. However, the dissenting minority report of Beatrice Webb and George Lansbury to the Royal Commission on the Poor Laws was in 1909 and foreshadowed the NHS. The all-UK Insurance Act of Lloyd George was in 1911 and provided medicine care for working men for the first time. These seem to me to be earlier and more radical ideas and law. Although the Lloyd George Act was not implemented until 1913 this was still before the First World War.' Letter to Ms Caroline Overy, 19 August 2016.

inquiry did was to describe things like rural poverty, the use of 'quack' American medicines, it made suggestions about making better use of technology, better use of the telephone, better use of the internal combustion engine, which was the thing of the day, but it made very important observations about rural generalism and the fact that the rural doctor was having to do many different things. They talked about access to rural services, to ambulances and getting into hospital, and made the first statements about the lack of access to what they called in those days 'postgraduate instruction'. So although there were qualified doctors and so on, they were not keeping up to date and they couldn't keep up to date because they couldn't get locums and they couldn't afford to pay locums while they went away and updated their knowledge. There was all the stuff there about teamwork, about the difficulty of obstetric care and the fact that there weren't enough midwives, so babies were dying; there were also poor immunization rates at the time. A whole number of different things and what they did in this report was that they tried to work out what would make things better. The doctors at the time said if only you gave us a small cottage hospital we could make things an awful lot better, if only we had a minimum income then we could do this properly. That was published in 1912 and it was accepted by the Government of the day.

What then happened was that the First World War came along and the Government of the day then spent all its money on blowing up Germans and it wasn't implemented. It didn't get implemented until around about 1923, and from that the concept of essentiality started and the idea that it was a human right, or a right in the UK for people, because they were deprived, because they were in poor conditions and so on, suffering from rural deprivation, they had a right to a medical service and the right to a midwife. This is where the concept of essentiality in the UK came from. Also, what happened was that because the people were too poor to pay for the service there was a fee-based structure all tied in with the 1911 National Insurance Act and so on that doctors were provided in those communities in the Highlands and Islands. What happened then was that the Highlands and Islands Medical Service started and began to function in the 1920s–1930s, and in the mid-1930s there was a government document in the UK called the Cathcart Report, which was the first beginnings of looking at whether there should be a national health service in the UK.[107] The Cathcart Report made direct reference to the Highlands and Islands Medical Service and, in fact, it was the first worked example of an on-the-ground, paid for, general

---

[107] Committee on Scottish Health Services (1936).

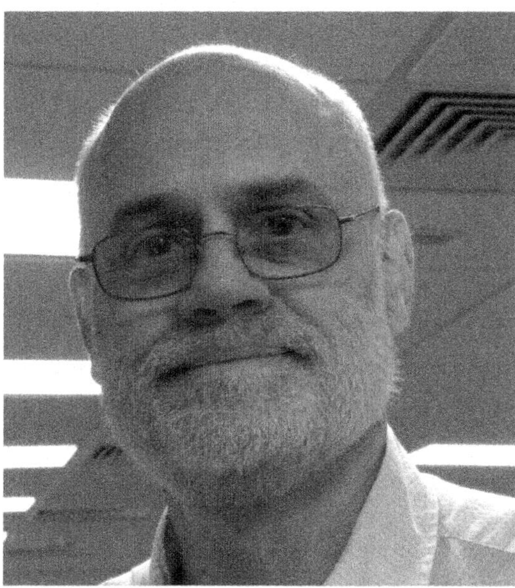

Figure 29: Professor Richard Hays

practitioner service in the UK. The Cathcart Report then went on to be one of the main documents, or main bits of thinking, behind the post-Second World War Government and the implementation of the National Health Service in 1948 in the UK.[108] The reason I'm going through this long introduction is that, in fact, you can date the establishment and the principles and the care of the NHS in 1948 in the UK right the way back to rural poverty in the Highlands and Islands of Scotland. It took decent qualitative modern methodology to define what the problems were, then to think of a solution, then for that solution to work in practice, then to say that's working very well, and then to implement it round the whole country. I think it's quite a good example where rural problems and rural innovation have then gone on to influence the big cities. That concept of the essentiality of general practice then became established throughout the whole of the UK, and I think that's a very important thing to celebrate as one of the successes of rural medicine and rural healthcare in the UK.

Professor Richard Hays: It might be worth just asking, to what extent do we want to look at the UK, which is where we're located, versus other models? Because, listening to what was said, there are obviously strong similarities with what's happened in Australia, and I suspect other parts of the world with a strong

---

[108] Further commentary on this point is provided by Professor Sir Denis Pereira Gray and has been archived with the records of this meeting (Wellcome Library, Archives and Manuscripts, GC/253).

British colonial connection, and yet there are very strong differences as well. Just to put that comment into context, I was a procedural rural doctor in Australia some years ago and that got morphed into rural medical education, initially running postgraduate training programmes for rural medicine in rural-orientated medical schools.[109] I'm from the northern part of Australia. North Queensland is actually quite different to the south and started off with a postgraduate rural programme and developed a highly integrated model. I then got seduced to the dark side of undergraduate medicine and became the founding Dean of James Cook University, which was the first new medical school for 26 years. It's founded on rural health and the Aboriginal health, and I recently went to the fifth graduation cohort party and they are in the cohort study that I'm still involved with, preferentially working in rural and regional Australia, which was the plan, so it does seem to work when you stack things up.[110] I then got seduced to England to set up what I was told was a rural medical school but I have discovered rural practice in England is a completely different kettle of fish. Nevertheless I've been working with the Institute of Rural Health in Wales and with John Wynn-Jones, whom many of us probably know. You will find in the main that Keele is doing some very radically different things in rural medical education, for England.[111] It wouldn't rate a ripple in the Australian headlines or in North America, but I think for England it will, and, in terms of academic training, my PhD is in educational psychology, my higher doctorate's in medical education, so lots of research and publishing around those things. I'm now going back to a more senior educational management role, having exited rural medicine, in a sense. I think the English regard general practice in Stoke-on-Trent as rural medicine, but there were several hundred thousand people there and that for me is a bit of stretch.

The concept of essentiality had not reached Australia in quite the same way as in the UK and it's a very different healthcare system, and yet the model of training and rural practice is almost certainly very similar to what began here. Even 25 years ago there had to be a strong need for procedural skills and that's still happening in much of Australia, and although it is declining, it's declined faster here. The concept of defining the practice population and the concept of how do you train for it, how do you keep your skills? There have been reports much

---

[109] For rural medicine in Australia in the 1980s, see Hays (2002).

[110] Hays, Stokes, and Veitch (2003); Hays, Veitch, and Lam (2005); Veitch, Underhill, and Hays (2006).

[111] Keele University School of Medicine was established in 2002 and developed its own undergraduate curriculum from 2007. See further discussion on pages 135–7, and comments by Professor Richard Hays on Keele Medical School in 2015 on page 39.

more recently in Australia. The ones I know very well were started around the mid-1970s when the Government suddenly realized they had a massive problem of mal-distribution of workforce and differences in healthcare outcomes – a lot of work has been done since then and Roger Strasser has been involved with a lot of that, as have I. The thing that strikes me though is that some of the people that I've come across in rural practice for the last 30 years in Australia fit into a discussion about 'quacks' and misfits – there were some remarkable characters out there who were slightly unusual and that's how they survived in rural medicine. There are lots of tales that could be told and some of them I had very direct experience with, but the history of it is, in a large sense, that of formal training for rural medicine and the true academic analysis of it is a post-Second World War phenomenon in Australia; up to that point there would have been an assumption that rural medicine was very similar.

Professor Roger Strasser: I'm also an Australian graduate, from Monash University, and I always thought I would become a rural general practitioner even as a student, and I tailored my postgraduate training in that direction, which in those days often included regular general practice training in Australia, coming to the UK and doing some extra house jobs in surgery and anaesthesia and the like. I came to Taunton in Somerset and was the senior house officer and Sarah was the houseman so that's how we met and one thing led to another, as you can probably gather. Just before I left Australia, I met some people from the University of Western Ontario and learned about the Master's programme they have, which is a training in academic family medicine. Having left Australia and being here in the UK, I thought while I was away from Australia maybe I would see if I could find my way into that programme, so I applied. Ian McWhinney[112] was the chair of the department at the time and somehow I managed to be accepted into that programme, so that's how we came to go to Canada after being here in the UK. I completed the Master's and then we both went back to Australia and joined a practice in a rural community called Moe, which is about two hours east of Melbourne in the south-eastern part of Australia in the state of Victoria. Having done the academic training, I had an interest, even as a student, in medical education and quite quickly I got involved in education and particularly the GP training programme. Having seen the GP training schemes here and the family medicine residency programmes in Canada I thought having a regional GP training scheme in Gippsland (which is that rural area in Australia) was a good idea, so I persuaded the local GP supervisors and the hospitals to buy into

---

[112] For Dr Ian Renwick McWhinney, see note 4.

this idea. We organized the rotations so that the trainees could actually do their GP training in Gippsland. This was at the time a new idea in Australia because GP training was organized on a state-by-state basis as a state-wide programme. Anyway, the programme was launched, however, it wasn't very well taken up by students and new graduates. In a sense that experience was what started me on the pathway that I'm still on today. Here was I and a number of colleagues in rural practice, very much enjoying it, but surprised to find that so few students and new graduates were interested in coming to join us. I started looking at the literature and then doing research and one thing led to another; it became clear that if this situation was going to change it needed to be addressed at the undergraduate level or even before the undergraduate level. An opportunity arose in 1991. Our local hospital and another hospital down the road were administratively amalgamated into a regional hospital and they had delusions of grandeur; they liked the idea of having an academic unit and so I put it to Monash University that they should have a rural academic unit. That was the beginning of what became the Monash University School of Rural Health.[113] I was appointed in 1992 as the first Professor of Rural Health, certainly in Australia and possibly in the world. One of the issues that clearly came forward was: 'If I'm a professor of rural health, what is the academic field? What is the discipline of rural health?' In 1994, certainly in retrospect, I put the cat among the pigeons by offering to present a paper at a joint meeting of the Royal New Zealand College of General Practitioners and the Royal Australian College of General Practitioners meeting in New Zealand. I was addressing the question 'Is rural practice a distinct discipline?' and that caused quite a stir.[114] The discussions about that are probably still going on today. Essentially, we developed the School of Rural Health with Monash University as a rural branch of the Metropolitan Medical School and by the time I left, it was a distributed network with four main centres and a network of other teaching sites providing clinical education for students in medicine, nursing, a range of other health disciplines (radiography, pharmacy, and so on), and also doing some research. In 2002 the opportunity came to go to Canada and to be involved in starting a multi-site, rural-based full medical school. So that's when I became the founding Dean of the Northern Ontario School of Medicine. I'm still in Canada as the Dean; the school took its first students in 2005 for a four-year graduate entry programme, so we had our first graduates in 2009.[115]

---

[113] See note 5.

[114] Strasser (1995).

[115] See note 6.

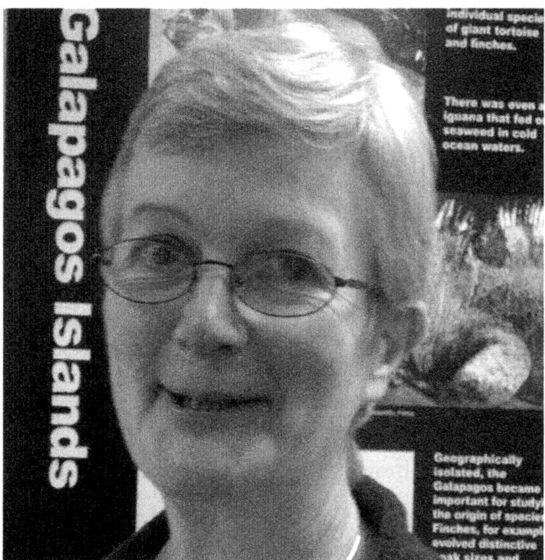

Figure 30: Professor Sarah Strasser

Professor Sarah Strasser: Perhaps I should just come in at this point? I'm a third-generation rural family doctor. My grandfather and parents were GPs in Penzance in Cornwall and my earliest memory was going with my grandfather to do visits out on the farms, and that's how I learned to ride a cow. I went to the Royal Free Hospital Medical School to learn medicine and that was an eye-opener in many ways. Having a lot of women as role models I never thought it was a problem until I got through medical school. I started my postgraduate training for family medicine, then general practice, in Cornwall, on the Isles of Scilly (1982–1983). I then married Roger and went west, went to Canada and completed my family medicine training under Ian McWhinney at the University of Western Ontario, and the second year in postgraduate training where we were taught about patient-centred medicine, but to me this was a normal course of events. We then went further west and lived in Australia for 18 years before returning to Canada, and since the 1990s have got more and more involved in medical education, in both postgraduate and undergraduate training, and it has required some drop in practice. I'm currently back in Sudbury (Laurentian University), with the key position of looking after third-year medical students who spend their whole year out in rural and remote practice on a guided apprenticeship model,[116] so that they are learning all of their objectives on the normal block rotation as well. They're actually based in general practice.

---

[116] Professor Roger Strasser added: 'The Comprehensive Community Clerkship in which students learn their core clinical medicine based in rural general practice. See Strasser *et al.* (2009) and Strasser *et al.* (2013).' Note on draft transcript 6 August 2016.

Pereira Gray: I think that sets the scene beautifully.

Roger Strasser: I was thinking of continuing the theme that Richard started and maybe suggesting that we are here in the UK and we're primarily focused on the history of rural medicine in the UK but also exploring the theme, particularly in the latter part of the twentieth century, of developments in different countries and then there's a feedback loop and certainly into this country. But on the theme of the genesis of rural medicine, as Jim [Douglas] suggested in the UK, in Australia there was a strong adherence and a belief in the value of generalism in medicine much later in the twentieth century than in this country. I think it's fair to say in this country that specialism had started to take over by the beginning of the twentieth century and that the specialists were concentrated in the hospitals and became consultants and started to differentiate from the role of GPs in the community; maybe started is not the right word. In Australia, even in the 1930s, the professors in specialist disciplines like obstetrics and gynaecology would actually be general practitioners who had a special interest in obstetrics and gynaecology, and even up until the 1950s new graduates in Australia went into practice, and it wasn't general practice, they went into practice. Then, as I heard it, those who didn't manage so well in practice then decided to narrow their field of medical practice and specialize. The change happened very quickly with the explosion of specialism and specialization in medicine. It happened elsewhere in the world and it certainly overtook Australia, so by the early 1970s, most new medical graduates were actually going straight into training to be a specialist and not into general practice. In the early 1970s the average age of general practitioners in Australia was going up by one year every year, in other words there were no graduates going into general practice. That was probably the main impetus for the Australian Government at the time to decide to fund general practice training. It started as a national programme delivered at state level in general practice. So that brings us to the 1970s and the question that's before us is: around when did rural medicine start?

Over the years, I knew a rural general practitioner, Robbie Fleming, in a town called Foster in South Gippsland. He started in practice in the early 1950s and was there for almost 50 years. He talked about how the scope of his practice changed in the 1970s. Until the 1970s, in his view, he and his medical colleagues – nursing staff, the local hospital, and so on – were able to provide the full range of medical services for common clinical problems to the people of Foster and the surrounding district as people would access in the city, in Melbourne, in the metropolitan area. Then, as he described it, it was in the 1970s with the rapid development of specialization and new technological developments and interventions in medicine, in his view, that they developed a separate pathway of rural medical practice in small communities compared to what happens in the larger urban centres.

Jim [Douglas] raised the theme of generalism and I think maybe the other question that's before us at the moment is what do we mean by rural medicine? I haven't mentioned WONCA, the World Organization of Family Doctors,[117] and we'll probably talk about the Working Party on Rural Practice at some stage,[118] but through that connection I think we've come to test and develop an understanding of rural medicine and rural practice pretty much around the world. It seems to be true to say that rural practitioners are extended generalists. When compared to their metropolitan counterparts, rural practitioners provide a wider range of services and carry a higher level of clinical responsibility in relative professional isolation. I think it's fair to say that that's true not only for doctors (and we're talking about GPs) but it's true actually for specialist physicians and surgeons and so on in rural regional centres, and true for nurses and pharmacists and physiotherapists and so on. What is rural medicine? It is doctors who have a broad generalist practice for whom there's a procedural element to their practice in some form, and as a general statement, dealing with emergencies is an unavoidable part of rural practice. The other element – and this is true for all rural practitioners in general but certainly for rural medical practitioners – is that there's a special community public health dimension to the practice. Rural practitioners have no choice but to live in the community they serve and so there's a relationship with the whole community that provides opportunities for affecting the health of the community at a whole community level. In the urban areas, these days, doctors often live in one part of the city and practise in another and so don't have that same opportunity. The ultimate is actually that the practice is in the home in terms of being a rural practitioner and so the whole family in a sense are rural practitioners and certainly living in a fishbowl.

Douglas: I want to go back to the history of the UK, because in the previous section I got us back as far as 1948 and the establishment of the NHS following the Dewar Report. Before that Will Pickles, a country GP in England, published his seminal *Epidemiology in a Country Practice*[119] when he was looking

---

[117] See note 7.

[118] See note 8.

[119] Pickles (1939). Dr William Pickles (1885–1969) was a GP in Aysgarth, Wensleydale, Yorkshire, for over 50 years; see Pemberton (1969).

at *Brucellosis* epidemiology, and he went on to be the founding President of the Royal College of General Practitioners. Again, I think that's a very fascinating example of a rural country doctor then influencing the whole system. If we then go on a little bit further, in the 1950s the BMA – the British Medical Association – produced a report on GP training[120] and in 1952 what we think is probably the first vocational training post or system was established in Inverness in Scotland. Inverness at that time was a small rural town and the concept was that a doctor would work in the local hospital and then work in the local general practice, and the whole concept of vocational training for general practice or family practice then became a movement within the UK and then started driving absolutely fundamental things in medical education in general. Certainly the whole vocational training movement, the Royal College of General Practitioners, patient-centred medicine, communication skills, etc., and the things that were developed in the vocational training during the 1960s and 1970s, then became integral; all the things about communication skills, teamwork, etc., then started driving medical education via the GMC (General Medical Council) in the UK in the 1980s, 1990s, 2000. Again, I think that that's an example where we can see the thread of things, maybe rural innovation starting then spreading as a wave going through the whole system.

If we're proceeding in the history of the UK then things started splitting up a little bit with the divergence of the health services around about 1999 when we had the devolution settlement in Scotland and the divergence of the health service system. Scotland was given the budget and told to run its own healthcare system in the same way as England, Wales, and Northern Ireland, and there are a number of papers that have been published recently looking back over the past ten years or so comparing these methods of state-run health service, how they differed.[121] One of the markers of healthcare in Scotland is that they have to provide services to remote islands – the Orkney Island, the Shetland Islands, the Western Isles, or remote communities within the land mass of Scotland – and so that's a challenge for the politicians. One of the things that now defines the health service in Scotland is the remote and rural issue and the safe delivery of healthcare. I was the project director for the Remote and Rural Areas Resource Initiative (RARARI) in Scotland in 2000, and started because of a review by the Chief Medical Officer at the time, Sir David Carter. He conducted the *Acute Services Review* and found that there was a problem in the surgical services – how

---

[120] British Medical Association (1950).

[121] See, for example, Greer (2008).

were they going to sustain hospital care in the Islands and the Highlands with increasing specialization of surgeons and maybe only one or two surgeons?[122] So then there became a whole programme in Scotland, because remote and rural healthcare is not just about general practice, it's also about how you provide the hospital side of the service without being consultant-led; should that be GPs with a particular interest? The whole political move towards increasing centralization has been a big challenge within devolved Scotland over the past ten years or so, and the debate has gone backwards and forwards between increasing medical technology, increasing specialization, and as things were getting costly therefore we had attempts to try to centralize everything but then the local public say no, no, we still have to have service locally and thus we have big dilemmas within remote and rural healthcare centred around that whole system debate. Again, I think now what is being found, certainly within Scotland, is that we're going back to the idea of the importance of generalism. Certainly, as we have an increasing changing demographic of society – we have an ageing and frail elderly population – it's now widely recognized that the answers to that are in good primary care and not getting old people into high-tech hospitals and doing inappropriate things to them. So I think that the whole circle is coming back round again to re-emphasizing the importance of strong and empowered primary care.

Dr Jim Cox: The question, when did rural medicine start, is an interesting one. There was an article in a newspaper last week talking about Stone Age man doing amputations and I guess that was rural medicine.[123] Until Victorian times, 1856 I think it was, England was predominantly a rural country; since that time it's become predominantly an urban country – I think that's England and not the UK; I'm not sure what the date is in Scotland. In 2009, last year, the world became predominantly urban, which is an interesting turning point.[124] Those demographics have obviously influenced healthcare and the way it's developed in this country. A major turning point was the introduction of the National Health Service in 1948. One way of looking at this is how rural healthcare has responded to the various challenges that have developed over the years.

---

[122] The acute services review was published in 1998: Scottish Office (1998). In 2000, the Remote and Rural Areas Resource Initiative (RARARI) was set up 'to develop healthcare services and support for professional staff in remote/rural parts of Scotland, funded by the NHS in Scotland … the organisation was disbanded on 31 March 2004': British Medical Association, Board of Science (2005), page 54.

[123] See, for example, Sage (2010); see also Buquet-Marcon, Charlier, and Samzun (2007).

[124] See page 58 and note 72.

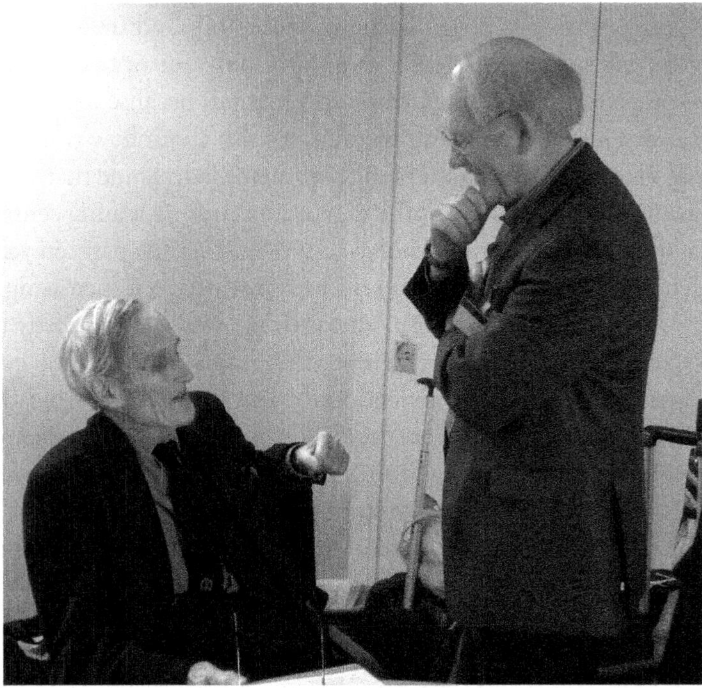

Figure 31: Professor Sir Eldryd Parry and Dr Jim Cox

The NHS is a curious organization in many ways: it is a national organization, but it is also a very local organization. What people expect is local delivery of healthcare, but it's a huge bureaucracy and the way that rural practices have responded has been different to the way that urban practices have responded, although the challenge is different in a small island where distances are generally much shorter. Nevertheless, rural doctors are responsible for their patients for very much longer; the patient can't go to hospital very quickly.

I began my career in the US in Springfield, Illinois, in the middle 1970s in a new medical school, which was set up to develop family medicine in the rural US,[125] and then was a GP in the Lake District until reasonably recently. In 1993 a letter from Gordon Baird to the Royal College of General Practitioners (RCGP) in London about a rural matter went all round the College and nobody knew who should deal with it until eventually it ended up with the 'Inner City Taskforce'. I was on Council of the College at the time and managed to rustle up enough interest to set up what was then called a rural practice group

---

[125] The Southern Illinois University School of Medicine was set up in 1970; for a brief history see www. siumed.edu/news/SIUhistory.htm (accessed 7 June 2016).

(it's now called a Rural Practice Standing Group).[126] We started that in 1993, stimulated, I have to say, by Gordon's letter I think. We spent the first few years trying to define what is different about rural healthcare in the context of a small country like the UK; it's different to Canada and Australia and New Zealand and the developing world with different needs, trying to kick off a literature in rural healthcare. Denis Pereira Gray was very helpful, as at the time he was the Honorary Editor of RCGP publications and he agreed to publish an occasional paper 'Rural General Practice in the UK'.[127] I'm currently working with the Commission for Rural Communities, an English body developed three or four years ago from the Countryside Agency, which is the Government's watchdog/ advocate and expert on rural matters – not particularly rural healthcare – in England, and I also work for the General Medical Council.

So how has rural practice responded to the different challenges? At the time of the beginning of the NHS one of the things that did affect rural practice was the separation of general practice from hospital practice and that's different to other countries. Most GPs don't have admitting rights to anything like a secondary care hospital; they may have access to smaller hospitals, which are changing. Specialist care has become much more sophisticated and much more effective, and the evidence for that is that the more procedures that are being done then the better the quality of care. So there's a strong argument on the one hand for centralization of services and yet you come back to the dilemma of the NHS – how do you provide a local service and at the same time balance access to services against quality of care? I think that's a constant underlying challenge for rural healthcare. One of the solutions (not a rural solution, but it has affected rural healthcare) is moving towards teamwork and towards substitution of care; other people doing jobs that GPs used to do.

Other big turning points in the 1990s and the early twenty-first century are the changes in the contract for GPs, and GPs no longer providing out-of-hours care.[128] That's produced huge challenges for everybody but it's also led to substitution. Other people are taking on the role of rural general practitioners;

---

[126] The Rural Forum replaced the Rural Practice Standing Group in November 2009. See Baird and Hogg (2010).

[127] Cox (ed.) (1995). Professor Sir Denis Pereira Gray added that he was, in particular, the Honorary Editor of the RCGP Occasional Papers, a series of academic monographs, which he introduced in 1976. Letter to Ms Caroline Overy, 19 August 2016.

[128] For a review of the provision of out-of-hours care in the mid-1990s, see, for example, Hallam (1994); and a later review by Grol, Giesen, and van Uden (2006).

part of that has been planned – nurse practitioners and out-of-hours healthcare providers – but part of it has been unplanned and that's been the ambulance service and accident and emergency departments in the secondary care hospitals. The ambulance service in particular has taken on a lot of primary healthcare. The point is that not all developments are planned; some of these things evolve. In terms of the care for patients, of course the ambulance service doesn't provide the same care that general practitioners can: there's no continuity, the default position is to take people to hospital and so on. I would urge us to look at this as a continuum and to look at the challenges that face rural healthcare now. Having said all that, we go back to Jim's [Douglas] starting point, which was, I think, that actually rural healthcare has in many ways led the way because it has been so much closer to patients and some of the traditions of rural general practice have been the traditions that people value most.

Pereira Gray: Thank you very much. We've had a pretty good run at the background and where it came from, and the history. I think we need to begin to think about the question of isolated practitioners as service providers: the problems and potentials and what level of provision? This is quite a sticky area so I think we need to look into that.

Dr Gordon Baird: I want to pick up Roger about the 1930s, because in fact in the 1930s there was no specialist maternity service in district general hospitals, and virtually all maternity care was general practice. I'm the third generation of general practitioners on the West Galloway and my grandfather, my father, and myself have covered all the local hospital provisions, including the maternity unit, the lifeboat, the military airfield, as well as private care in general practice. I have been heavily involved in training general practitioners and students on a personal level for nearly 30 years now. Against the advice of my father and uncle and many colleagues and probably my grandfather if he had been alive, I got involved (and don't particularly regret it) with Jim Cox as a founder member of the Rural Practice Standing Group of the Royal College. I have to say we're still struggling with a College that appears to care less than it should about rural primary care, and I think that it has much to learn from rural health and much more to gain than it has to lose from engaging with this subject, but that is a big struggle currently. I have to say this when I'm down in London – it's a big struggle for us at the periphery with the increasing power of the College and I think that represents our biggest challenge for the future, because I think we'll go on to that.

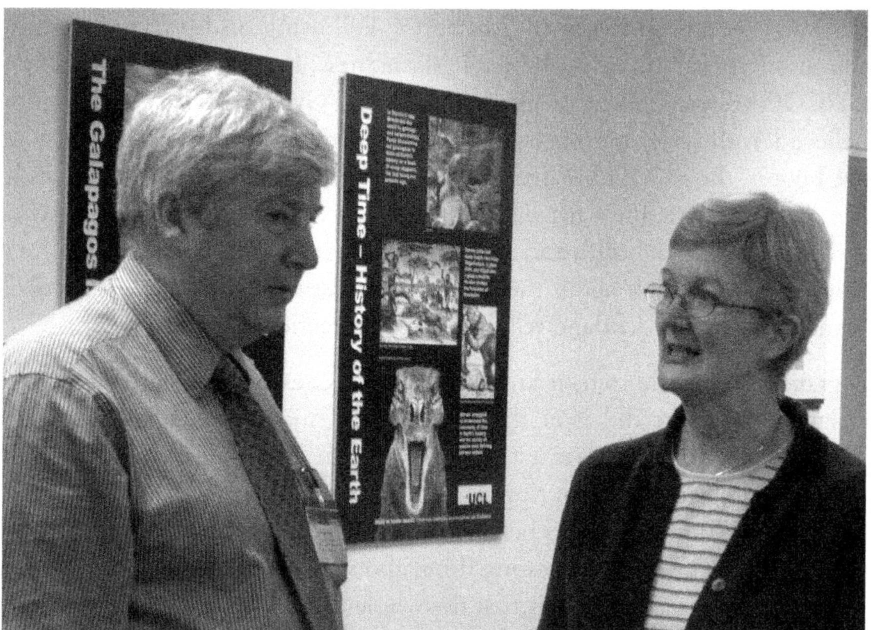

Figure 32: Dr Gordon Baird and Professor Sarah Strasser

It's a pleasure to see Jim Douglas and Iain McNicol here, because we were involved with RARARI, which was important and significantly contributed to the research base for rural primary care in Scotland.[129] I think Jim ought to be congratulated, because what he did was visionary and took a considerable personal toll; I'm proud to have been associated with that. I continue, for the moment, until I get Jim and Iain's job, to continue as a GP and a family doctor but also as a hospital practitioner, having moved away from a part-time post to being a fairly full-time hospital practitioner in our community hospital and I am clinical lead for the hospital, which deals with 1,400 acute medical admissions a year.[130] There is a maternity unit there, which is now midwife-led but when it was GP-led, I published in the *BMJ* about that.[131] We were the first GPs in the UK to routinely deliver thrombolysis for myocardial infarction based at our community GP-led hospital,[132] and they have just become the first community-based unit to deliver thrombolysis for acute stroke. I also published the first

---

[129] See pages 96–7.

[130] The Galloway Community Hospital, Stranraer.

[131] Baird, Jewell, and Walker (1996).

[132] Gordon (1989).

descriptions of Lyme disease in Scotland.[133] Following on from my maternity publication, it might have been in a fit of madness, I passed the Membership of the RCOG (Royal College of Obstetricians and Gynaecologists) examination. I believe I'm the only person to have achieved this from general practice and since I got it, the RCOG has decided that GPs are not allowed to apply for this exam; I'm not quite sure what that says about me. My current interests include deprivation and rural health and access to secondary and tertiary care; again I've published a bit on that about the very poor access to tertiary care, particularly of cancer patients in Scotland relating to rural practice.[134]

My grandfather is said to have arranged the first Caesarean section in Dumfries in Galloway and he did it at the request of a midwife and he phoned the ambulance, arrived at the same time, stopped the train at Glenwhilly station, the train waited for the labouring woman who was transferred up to Glasgow to the Western Infirmary and I believe that both were safe and well at the end of the procedure. The most interesting thing about that when talking about access to secondary and tertiary care is that the whole thing took less than four hours. If we currently call a helicopter, the mean time to hospital is between four and a quarter and four and a half hours, and I think that is what is called progress. [Laughter] I guess what we have lost – and I agree with what Jim's saying – is that GPs, particularly in rural areas, were part of the social capital, part of the social framework; they belonged. Even those succumbing to alcohol through isolation and perpetual on-call were belonging and tolerated, because they were part of the social framework and overall they did more good than harm, in the main. I think the disaster of the Thatcher years, and subsequently, is the commodification of medicine. I would like to think that rural practice can still lead the profession out of that commodification of medicine and healthcare because that is its worst and desperate aspect. I feel we've still got some of that in rural practice, and I feel that much can be learned from the past.

Dr Iain McNicol: As a genuinely remote practitioner, maybe I can fill in some of the problems that we've seen and some of the changes that have happened to talk about isolated practitioners. I'm a recently retired GP from Port Appin in Argyll.

---

[133] Dr Gordon Baird elaborated: 'Later we also broke new ground when we diagnosed a new presentation of Lyme disease in a patient who had the diagnosis missed at several teaching hospitals. This was followed by a practice based serological study demonstrating that Lyme disease exposure was common in dairy farmers: Bourke *et al.* (1988), Baird *et al.* (1989).' Email to Ms Caroline Overy, 15 November 2016; see also the comments on Lyme disease by Dr James Douglas on page 34.

[134] Baird *et al.* (2008).

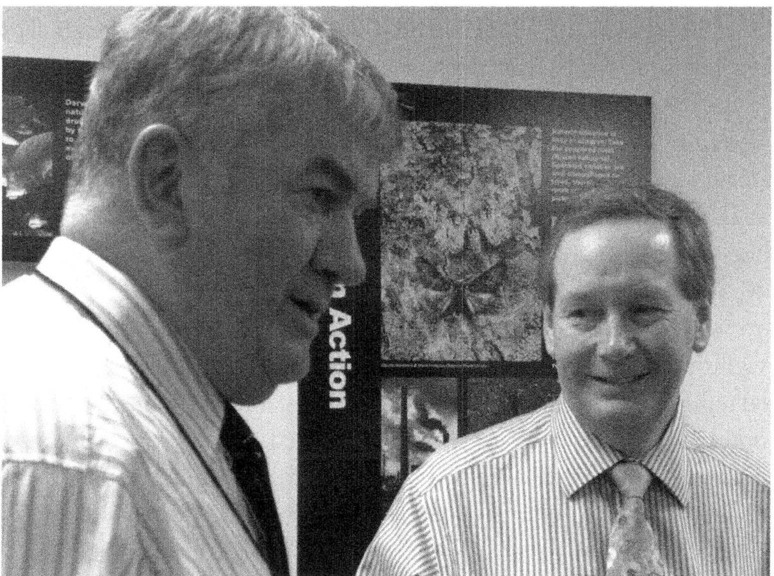

Figure 33: Dr Iain McNicol and Dr James Douglas

I've been there for 30 years, taking over from my father in the same practice. I did my postgraduate education in the Memorial University of Newfoundland and did a two-year residency in remote and rural practice, which was the first one in the world at the time.[135] I practised in the Orkney Islands for a couple of years before coming to Appin. I was chair of Scottish BASICS[136] for a while and was involved in setting up the Pre-hospital Immediate Care Training Scheme in Argyll and throughout Scotland. I've been a tutor at Aberdeen University, Queen's University at Kingston, Ontario, and I did 12 years of an exchange with Middlebury College of Vermont on educating children to see whether they wanted to do medicine, straight-A students going into medicine and trying to weed out the 35 per cent who wouldn't do it.[137]

After the health service came in in the UK there was a scheme called Inducement Practices Scheme in Scotland, which basically, where essentiality was concerned, guaranteed minimum salary, which was 80 per cent of the UK GP average. With

---

[135] See comments by Professor James Rourke on Memorial University on page 16.

[136] BASICS is a national organization, formed in 1977, which runs courses in cardiac and trauma resuscitation to provide emergency, on-scene, pre-hospital care. Scottish BASICS was set up in 1993 with the demand for courses in remote regions; the organization registered as a charity, BASICS Scotland, in 2002; see http:// basics-scotland.org.uk/ (accessed 16 May 2016).

[137] See further discussion on this project on page 132.

the Robinson changes in 1965,[138] which did a lot to improve general practice with ancillary staff in central premises, inducement practice fell way behind because they were basically working from the house, as has been described, and I certainly remember that well. By 1973 we set up an association called the Inducement Practices Association, which I chaired for many years and in fact I'm the Life President of the Remote Practitioners' Association now.[139] In those days we got 21 days paid leave per annum and we worked 344 days a year, 24/7. We were paid 80 per cent of the UK national average and had none of the access to services that the Robinson Report had brought in. So we campaigned fairly vigorously and by 1990 a whole lot of dramatic things happened that changed remote practice. The Associate Scheme came in thanks to Dr Somerled Fergusson who worked hard for it, which allowed one doctor to share between three practices and give 17 weeks a year relief to each practice.[140] Quickly that was extended in fact to one between two so that made a huge change in what happened. The second thing was the Scottish Ambulance Helicopter Service became available for the first time and so there was the possibility of getting help for the seriously ill and the injured. I agree with Gordon, you can wait a long time for a helicopter, but the principle was there. I mean the retrieval achieved now from Glasgow is tremendous and that has raised standards and is part of supporting remote practice. The third thing that happened in the late 1980s was the Lockerbie bomb. That was a total disaster for the Scottish Ambulance Service, luckily nobody suffered for it, because there was nobody to suffer, but 49 single-manned ambulances turned up at Lockerbie and I think there was one two-manned ambulance.[141] It totally embarrassed the Scottish Ambulance Service, it embarrassed the Scottish Home and Health Department at that time, and they looked at things very hard and, directly because of that, money was given to rural practice to start pre-hospital, immediate care training

---

[138] Sir Kenneth Robinson (1911–1996) was Minister of Health from 1964 to 1968 in the Labour Government under Harold Wilson. His negotiations led to the Family Doctors' Charter agreed by the Government in 1965 and which came into effect in 1966. New contracts encouraged GPs to expand their practices, employing healthcare teams and improving their premises: British Medical Association (1965).

[139] The Inducement Practices Association became the Remote Practitioners' Association and then in 2014 was renamed the Rural GP Association of Scotland (RGPAS); http://scotland.ruralgp.com/ (accessed 16 May 2016).

[140] For a discussion of the Associate Scheme see, for example, Marshall (1997).

[141] In December 1988, Pan Am flight 103, en route from London to New York, was blown up over the Scottish town of Lockerbie; all 259 passengers and 11 people on the ground were killed.

and the whole thing came from Lockerbie.[142] Double manning in ambulances became the standard and so a lot of the infrastructure and the support in remote practice, which we've been talking about other professionals, began to be put in place at that time.

A couple of things on literature which I'm not sure if you've got is *Single-handed* was produced in 1988, it was funded by RARARI eventually in 2002 and that was done because single-handed practice was seen to be disappearing.[143] John Bain, a professor of general practice in Dundee, and Rosie Donovan, a photographer, went round 47 of us and stuck a microphone in front of us and took a picture and said, 'Talk', and they analysed that, so that was a qualitative review of single-handed practice and a good historical basis. When I was working with Vermont, I showed them that book, in fact I gave each student a book and Vermont produced their own version of it called *Caring for our Own*, which is a broader thing, it talks to community OTs, community physiotherapists, patients as well as doctors, and that's the Vermont rural aspect of things, so there are a couple of literature things that do exist.[144] In 2004 the new contract, of course, the idea of essentiality has been removed and we did think we'd see a lot of remote practice disappear, but the Government hasn't had the nerve so far to do it so communities are hanging on to their own because politicians are saying why fight with a thousand people unnecessarily? But the essentiality has gone, in the new contract.[145]

Sarah Strasser: Might I just say, my perspective of the UK is from when I can start remembering until I left in the early 1980s, despite a few visits back since. I was just thinking about the differences and liked the idea of perhaps looking at defining a practice population. I'm sure that the NHS coming in must have made a huge change. My recollection of my grandfather was that he knew everyone for generations and generations and everyone knew him and he was always greeted wherever we went. In Cornwall – I'm sure they were as poor as they were in Scotland – payment came by chickens or eggs or whatever and that seems to have changed quite a bit, along with the nature of the gift. I

---

[142] Steedman *et al.* (1991).

[143] Donovan and Bain (eds) (2000).

[144] Bellerose (2006).

[145] For the details of the 2004 contract, see Department of Health (2003). The legislation introduced in 2004 is available online at www.legislation.gov.uk/uksi/2004/291/pdfs/uksi_20040291_en.pdf (accessed 18 May 2016). For the impacts of the new contract, see for example, Peckham (2007).

remember that one of the gifts we had was that I would go on holiday to one of the local farmers and pitch up a tent in their field and a girl that was roughly my age got polio and I would go and visit her in her iron lung. I'm sure there's all these wonderful descriptions that could be a part of our corporate memory if people's memories are better than mine anyway. But things like knowing generations of families have gone and it got me thinking about perhaps having some of these memories of the past and seeing what is very different with that.[146] The other thing that was mentioned was about GPs not having visiting rights; well, I remember my grandfather and my parents, regardless of whether they had visiting rights or not, they felt it was their duty to visit their patients in hospital and if they had small children around their ankles off we went too. In fact, I would say – and I tell this to my students now – when you refer your patient to the obstetrician that's when they need you most. House calls were a fantastic thing and you got to see a patient out of the clinic setting, out of your room setting, which gave you a totally different dimension of how that person was functioning and coping with their illness.

Roger Strasser: I think that one of the themes here is the closeness of the rural practitioner, particularly in the isolated setting, to the whole community, as we've heard, and maybe even though with the removal of essentiality it's that sense of being part of the community and responding to the need of the community. It seems to me that a key issue here for people in the small communities is about access to care, and the local GP, nurses, and other health providers are the frontline providers of that care. You talked about the ambulance service and evacuation and so on; I think that one of the critical issues is actually the same for people wherever they are, that is, that people anywhere, whether in the city or in the rural and remote areas, have a security need. They need to know that if they are unlucky enough to be seriously ill or injured that the system is there to save them; that there's a safety net provided by the system and they look to the doctor and the nurse or whoever. They certainly value having a hospital and somehow assume that if there's a hospital that that safety net is there for them. You talked about a small island; I suppose you were meaning the UK? Because, of course, when you're talking about islands, I was thinking of John MacLeod and his career as a GP and his father before him in North Uist in

---

[146] Professor Sir Denis Pereira Gray added: 'I agree with Sarah that knowledge of generations of families has greatly reduced but it is not quite accurate to say that it has "gone". Certainly as late as 2000, I measured 7% of my whole practice list having a four generation relationship with me and in a city practice in Exeter and I knew them personally and their relationships.' Letter to Ms Caroline Overy, 10 November 2016.

the Outer Hebrides.[147] That's a small island and that's remote, especially in bad weather and with really challenging communications. One of the realities of rural living and rural practice is that you have small populations, large distances, challenging terrain, often difficulties with communication and transportation, limited resources – financial resources and human resources – and so it's a matter of making the best with what is available. It also means that the service delivery models that you have, which work in a small rural or remote community, are different from the service delivery models that work in the urban areas. Talking about policy issues, we keep coming back to policy like the NHS coming out of an earlier report and so on; one of the problems is that so often policy decisions are made in the metropolitan area and they're addressing issues that are concerns in the big urban centres and often have unintended and unrecognized negative consequences in rural areas. I remember when I visited John MacLeod once after devolution, I said to him, 'Well, how is it? It must be better now you've got a Scottish Government?' and he said actually it was worse, because he said that the people in London knew that they didn't know anything about North Uist, but the people in Edinburgh think they do know about North Uist. [Laughter]

Hays: Isolation is a fascinating concept and I'd like to start off by saying some of the most isolated practitioners I've met have been in large cities, so official isolation is not just about distance and rurality. In fact, much of the success of rural medicine in Australia has been because, as a rule, rural doctors are very well networked and know how to communicate with each other, and actually they're better at communicating with the Government quite often than their urban counterparts. But back at the level of isolation, I reflect upon my time in the early 1980s as a rural doctor, so at one stage I was one of four doctors in a town of about 10,000, there were four ambulance bearers who only ever went out one at a time and I can remember occasions where I'd get a phone call: 'There's been a road accident 80 miles up the road, mate, can you come with me, because I can't drive and deal with it?' So I'd call one of the other GPs and say: 'Can you look after the hospital for four hours?', because that's how long it took and I'd be haring up there. I remember at one stage, because the ambulance driver had better skills at resuscitation than I, we swapped roles, so I was driving the ambulance at 80 miles an hour down this road, literally dodging kangaroos at dusk – it's very dangerous in that respect – while the ambulance driver took on the role at the back. In a sense I don't look upon my time as a rural doctor as being particularly isolated because I worked quite comfortably

---

[147] For Dr John MacLeod see page 35 and note 40.

with a team of people around me and that's one of the key points that, in fact, I believe rural practitioners, of all professionals, actually are pretty happy to blur the boundaries a bit, work together, give and take, share call after hours.[148]

It's interesting that a lot of these new substitution models don't necessarily seem to be designed to work as teams; there seem to be additional people that do particular roles, and one of the things that's happened, at least in Australian roles, is that it's had to be defined by what it needs to do rather than what others have taken off. There was an interesting fight back in the 1990s and the 2000s about that.[149] In a sense while Australia is going to produce physician assistants (PA) on the US model, it's been absolutely unclear what role they will play and will they take roles off nurses and doctors and how will they relate to nurses and doctors? The professional isolation, there are some one-doctor towns in northern Australia where I worked, where on reviewing the community development models, as academics, we decided the only way to fix this town, to stop it losing burned-out doctors every two or three years was to find enough money to make it a two-doctor town or to put in another layer so people could share all the work. I've got a PhD student at the moment who's done a series of case studies that's about to be submitted, where they found a remote area nurse station has exactly the same professional isolation and burnout problems as the remote area silo GP model.

I think the sensible thing to do is to look upon professional isolation as not a uni-profession or uni-discipline thing. It's about putting a team out there as well. In northern Australia we found some towns could never support health professionals, they were very demanding, whereas others were lovely stable places where the people became part of the healthcare team and worked very collaboratively with the doctors and nurses, etc., and the visiting people. So, teamwork there is not just about medicine, it's about other professions, it's also about the community in partnership with their healthcare providers in making it work, and that overcomes an awful lot of isolation. It's something we did at James Cook University – when students went to rural placements the first thing they did was they met the mayor and the local councillor, they put on a

---

[148] See Hays (2002).

[149] Professor Richard Hays wrote: 'At the time there was disagreement between nurse practitioners and medical practitioners about the potential roles of physician assistants (PA), and also concerns amongst some medical practitioners that physician assistants might reduce employment for junior doctors. It did not reach any public level, but one result was that very few PA positions were created and the then main PA degree programme (Queensland University) was closed.' Email to Ms Caroline Overy, 12 July 2016.

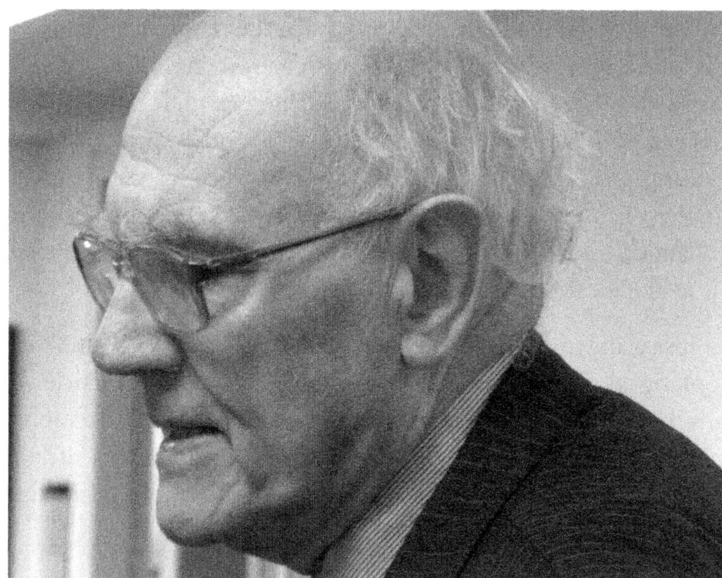

Figure 34: Professor Sir Denis Pereira Gray

barbecue for them down at the local lake or the river; we attached students to a community rather than to practices and we were very careful about that.[150] Maybe that comes more under education later.

Pereira Gray: I'm very conscious that the room is full of people who've got enormous lifetime experiences and who are hugely dedicated and have got a great deal to be proud of. I want to confront what's just been said about the loss of essentiality, and I think for the UK people here there is this huge impact of a time-limited contract. To sharpen it up, I come from Exeter, there's a story that's talked a lot about now in my part of the world about a village not very far from Exeter, about 20 miles away, where on a Saturday morning a kid got mild asthma and the GP's answerphone said ring NHS Direct, which is a national telephone centre.[151] So what then happens is that a nurse in Bristol, which is 100 miles away, sends an ambulance to this child and then drives it to my local hospital, where the child gets put on a nebulizer and is sent home, passing the rural GP who was mowing the lawn at the time and for 200 years would have dealt with that locally. I don't want to be awkward but I think we have to

---

[150] See comments by Professor Richard Hays on pages 38–9.

[151] NHS Direct was set up in 1998 as a 24-hour telephone-based advice and information service in England and Wales. In England, it was discontinued in 2014 and the NHS 111 service was set up as the 24-hour non-emergency NHS number.

confront today some of the huge implications in the new contract, which means that the GP doesn't regard himself as serving his local community, he's 'off duty' was the word that's been used here and also the fact that the ambulance cost £250. I happen to have contacts at national level and I know that that sort of story is causing great anger and repercussions because it's perceived as a gross waste of money. I think it's something about the way medicine has changed; it's certainly changed the attitude of that village to doctors plural and it's certainly changed it to the local GP mowing his lawn.

I think we just want to come a little bit into the sharp end – is this sustainable? Are we looking at a huge change in the nature of rural practice? Is a 250-year culture being shattered? Is this retrievable? Are we going to solve it with telemedicine? I think a little bit more of the sharp edge and a little bit more about the technological alternatives that people in London are talking about, metropolitan though they may be.

Douglas: Can I say, I'm a rural doctor, I still do on-call and I run our local out-of-hours service, and I still get out of my bed in the middle of the night to go and see people. The reason that I do that is that I was involved when the new contracts were set up and if there was to be any service somebody had to do it, so I tried to keep everybody onboard locally to provide a service. What we did do was that from our rural town of Fort William, by better use of technology, with a car and a driver and better use of mobile phone technology, etc., we extended our range of cover so that we covered some of the smaller practices that were then looking pretty unviable in terms of the two-doctor practices and being forever on-call. I think the sensible extension of out-of-hours service, certainly within remote and rural Scotland, has preserved the viability of GPs in smaller communities. There is the difficult question about where do you actually draw the line? We've extended that line and there are still several practices where there is no other solution, that I can see anyway, apart from having a very skilled generalist onsite, on the ground, such as Iain's practice just down the road from me; such as some of the small islands; such as the geographical islands, if you like, on mainland Scotland. That's all about a perception of community safety, community resilience, that people have talked about and the importance of that. I think there is an important thing about having the most skilled personnel. There's a paradox here that if you're a major incident medical officer, as I am, if there's a major incident in my area I'm the person that trots out to the bus crash or the train crash or whatever and does the triage on scene. The principle of triage is you want your most experienced person at the site of the bus crash; if it's a hospital triage you have your most experienced physician or surgeon standing on the door of the hospital, not stuck in the theatre. I think when people were talking about the make-up of teams and 'Can you delegate some of this to nurses and paramedics?' and all the rest, there comes a point, for all sorts of reasons – either because it's confidence, because it's skill mix, retention of skills, the number of times you see things, all these sorts of things – when, in fact, you do need the most competent generalist, and that should probably be, in certain circumstances, the doctor; there are things that you can't delegate.

Rural generalism, I think, probably has to be medical practitioners in certain remote communities, but those remote practitioners do need support. We can support people now through the new generation, people like David [Hogg] with the internet, chat rooms, we have video conferencing, etc., and most of us are very confident. I'm very confident with video conferencing and using technology, despite being 'an older doctor'. If we are thinking about the strength of rural communities, one of the assets of rural medicine is the visibility of problems. One or two people have already referred to this and I want to draw this as one of the strengths of rural practice – if you're within a community you can see things happening. You know the patients; in my own case, for instance, a new industry comes into my local town, people start getting asthma when they didn't have asthma before, therefore I do a research project to prove that this factory is causing asthma in those particular patients.[152] That's because things are visible and because I can see them and because I'm part of the whole and that's one of the strengths also of medical education that Roger and Richard have been talking about in rural areas. In other words, certainly in my area, it's very easy to join other parts of the whole. We have a junior doctor working at the local hospital who then comes and works in my local practice and then we can get them to see and triangulate their care of seeing the patient at the practice and also working in the hospital and joining up the bits, so it's the whole thing about visibility and understanding.

I think when we're asking, 'Well, what can rural bring? How can we maybe re-establish some of the traditional values?', there's a great importance in trying to maintain and sustain the traditional values of rural healthcare, rural general practice to help solve some of the problems of the twenty-first century that we see before us. I think these are very serious and challenging problems about preserving rural identity, giving rural professional people a status and feeling

---

[152] See note 153, and Dr James Douglas' comments on page 34.

empowered, and feeling that they're just as good as the people in the big cities. The people in the big cities are actually now admitting that we're also specialists. They recognize that they only understand one very narrow bit of medicine or one very narrow bit of surgery and they now want the complete generalist, and the only generalists left are basically general practitioners or people with general practitioner training. In Scotland we are beginning to go the full circle, and the physicians are now saying that for the acute medical wards we want people who have been through general practice training and we give them more training.

Pereira Gray: Thank you very much. Just for the record, James had an important article in the *Lancet* in the 1990s on the outbreak of asthma in his practice, which turned out to be due to a local fishing factory, and that's a very good example of a local practice solving a local problem by onsite research.[153]

Dr David Hogg: I want to make an observation, particularly picking up the impact of the cultural changes that are happening in the UK, about the impact of that on trainees and also the impact on patients. I'm actually a GP registrar from Kilmarnock, which is not so much of a rural location, however, I'm very interested in going into rural practice eventually. Last year I represented 500 West of Scotland trainees on the RCGP Trainees' Committee and partly because of that I became a trainees' representative on the newly formed RCGP Rural Forum. I also run a blog 'Rural GP', which I understand is one of the reasons that I've been asked to attend today, so although I don't bring huge amounts of experience, I hope I bring enthusiasm and I'm fascinated to hear what's going on today; thank you for inviting me.[154]

First of all: the impact on trainees, particularly in terms of unscheduled care, along with the idea that you are supposed to clock off at 5 o'clock because of the EU Working Time Directive and you're chased off by a manager with a big stick if you don't, because you're not allowed to stay on later. I'm a trainee who's gone through that system, and the European Working Time Directive has affected a lot of my training, perhaps eroding the initial senses that are instilled in you in medical school, such as the Hippocratic Oath – of your being there as a trustworthy doctor who will go to whatever length it takes to provide

---

[153] Douglas *et al.* (1995).

[154] Since 2013, Dr David Hogg has been a GP partner in the Arran Medical Group, and is editor of RuralGP.com, a resource set up in 2009 'for remote & rural GPs, GP trainees and nurses. It aims to provide up-to-date information about key events, discussions and initiatives for UK rural general practice'; http://ruralgp.com/ (accessed 23 May 2016).

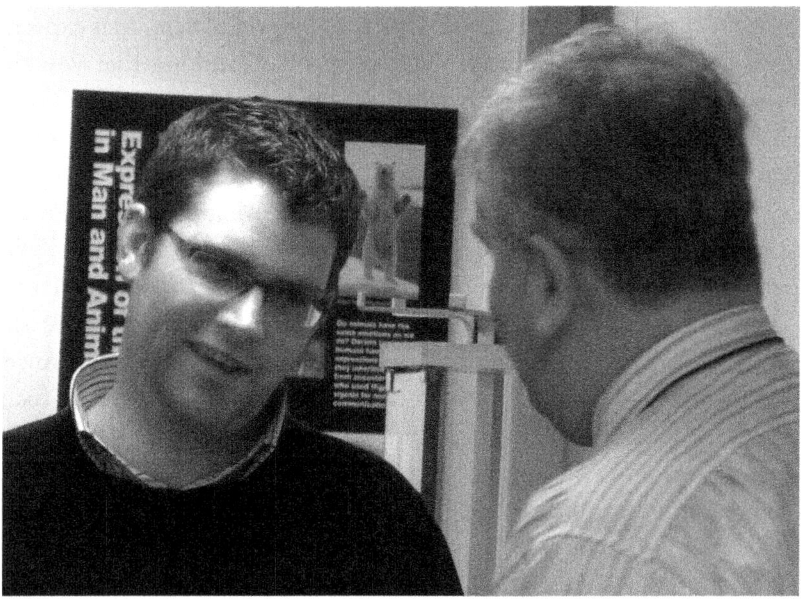

Figure 35: Dr David Hogg and Dr Iain McNicol

patients with good care. As someone coming through the current system of training it sets up the expectation in trainees that this more restrictive method of working practice will always be in place and, as I say, it does erode the sense of duty that goes with the job. I think on the flipside I would like to think that those individuals who want to go into rural practice acknowledge that these restrictions aren't so dogmatic; trainees who want to go into rural practice are those who certainly do want to preserve a large sense of that duty, who want to continue that and who aren't scared by the idea of being on call all the time. The major challenge to that, however, is the changing culture fostered by NHS 24 and NHS Direct in patients.[155] As patients become more familiar with 'it doesn't matter if I phone someone at 3 o'clock in the morning because I'll get through to a call centre where there are nurses standing by there waiting for me', it's very difficult to change that culture, and so I certainly agree that there needs to be a certain brake applied to some of the changes going on if we are to preserve some of the 24-hour local services, which are available to patients in rural areas.

My own feeling now is that one of the major challenges that defines rural practice, and which as a trainee is helping me to understand that, is the growth of specialisms. The growing specialization and centralization of care and how

---

[155] Launched in 2002, NHS 24 is an online and out-of-hours telephone service providing 24-hour health advice to people in Scotland: www.nhs24.com/ (accessed 23 May 2016). For NHS Direct see note 151.

patients have been encouraged to expect a certain level of care, that expectation has been driven largely by the inequalities agenda, thinking that you should be able to access the same services whether you're living next to the Southern General Hospital in Glasgow or in a remote area, for example the Isle of Lewis. It's great to have that aspiration, everyone has that same access to standards of care, however, realistically that is never going to happen and I think that people who actually realize that are mostly the patients who are in rural practice and particularly the GPs in rural practice. It's about how you can impress those conflicting expectations of 'we pay our taxes and therefore we should have exactly the same access to care', whereas it's not possible to provide it. Increasingly now we're coming away from evidence-based practice and focusing more on the patient's experience and actually delivering evidence-driven decisions. For example, translation of guidelines, which can be implemented in large centralized centres of care, but aren't always best for every patient. If you're 60, 70, 80, if you're particularly frail, a journey down to Glasgow by helicopter could have serious health disadvantages, whereas if you can be cared for somewhere more locally that's far superior in terms of that person's welfare.

Baird: I agree with the NHS 24 comments, which was, of course, from my perspective, imposed on our community. My wife used to answer the phone for nothing for many years, as did my mother; when the on-call was centralized to a system within our casualty department it was £6 to £12 per call and NHS 24 now costs £36 to £60 per call, simply for the call handling. The trade-off for that was an increase in call-outs for the GPs. NHS 24 caused a fourfold increase in home visits, there was a similar increase in ambulance call-outs and when we challenged them that they were four times as expensive and four times worse, they said: 'Well, we're going to get better.' I asked: 'How much better?' and they said: 'Well, we should reduce that by half.' I said: 'So then you'll only be twice as bad' and they were extremely resentful about that. While I can understand their resentment, I'm appalled that they couldn't understand my position and the problem is the difference between locally developed versus centrally imposed systems. If there's a lesson to be learned from history, throughout this, it is that locally developed systems outperform centrally imposed systems in rural areas and that is the big, big message. I do not miss the on-call, however. There was a locum who came to work in our practice once and had been at this single-handed practice the week before. He was absolutely shattered and terrified at the morning surgery because on two days in a row he'd had a myocardial infarction presenting and it wasn't an appointment system; the patient attended the waiting room, waited in the queue and stumbled into his surgery clutching his chest, the second of which arrested. They were not discouraged by their GP who they'd been calling but they knew this single-handed GP was relentlessly on-call and, being decent folk, they did not want to disturb him. So I guess we need to seek a balance somewhere, but what I am convinced of, personally, is that the balance of these centrally developed, centrally imposed, centrally run systems has gone too far in the wrong direction and I don't believe that it is or ever will be, however well run, a complete solution for rural areas.

Cox: It's interesting to hear from David Hogg. I don't know how much you want to talk about the future or how much we're supposed to be talking only about history. One of the difficulties is that both patients and, to a certain extent, doctors want it both ways and I think you've highlighted that, Denis, with your anecdote. What patients want is a traditional service where their doctor will attend them at any hour of the day or night – that's not a rural phenomenon and many urban practices have provided very personal care. I can't refer to any particular evidence, but I'm pretty sure it's true that it has sustained longer in rural communities where the local doctor is visible, he's embedded in the community. Even if the surgery's no longer in the doctor's house, the home is still part of the community in remote and many rural practices. There's this sense of responsibility and then a willingness to improvise when things get awkward or difficult, to think outside the box a bit, and we experienced this to a huge extent during the foot and mouth outbreak in 2001 where we did all sorts of strange things. I remember reducing somebody's dislocated shoulder at a farm gate because they weren't allowed out of the farm and I wasn't allowed in. I was dealing with quite seriously ill people in the back of cars for the same reason.[156] The 'solution', as Gordon says, has predominantly been policy driven from the centre. The solution for the problem of individual practices and doctors not being able to provide 24-hour care because of increasing demand has worked differently in urban than in rural areas. I don't think it works in urban areas either, but it certainly doesn't work in rural areas and it needs rethinking. The times are wrong. From a patient's point of view, it's quite absurd, particularly if there's more than one doctor, that they're available at the same time and then off duty at the same time. This Saturday morning business, for example, doesn't make any sense to patients at all. Again, it comes to a balance: how do you balance increasing patient demand and the European Working Time Directive changing the work culture in junior doctors with the strong sense

---

[156] See comments regarding isolation during the 1967 outbreak of foot and mouth disease at the Witness Seminar on that outbreak, in Reynolds and Tansey (eds) (2003), 34–6.

of professional people wanting to provide the best professional service that they can? One thing that's clearly not going to work, because it was one of the tenets of the NHS but has never worked, was the expectation that by providing free universal healthcare that the amount of ill health would diminish and it would become cheaper and demand would go down. People still talk about it, extraordinarily, but clearly it doesn't work. It's not going to work and nobody has worked out a way of reducing demand. It's not going to happen.

Roger Strasser: David talked about people wanting to be cared for locally, in my estimation that is one of those realities of the rural setting and the necessities for rural healthcare. In almost 20 years in rural practice in Australia, twice I had people who chose to go blind rather than travel a couple of hours to the nearest ophthalmology service. It's interesting you triggered this line of discussion with the story about asthma. One of my issues in talking about 'rural versus urban' is the different meaning of the same word. A hospital in the big city is this huge monolithic intimidating de-personalizing institution that you want to stay out of if you possibly can, and in a small rural community the hospital – I guess in the UK it would be a cottage hospital – is actually almost a 'home away from home'. The staff are known as friends and family members and so on. The story that highlights this occurred in a small rural community in Australia. There'd been some consternation because they were looking at hospital admission rates for asthma and the high-profile asthma specialist, the respiratory specialist at the Royal Children's Hospital in Melbourne, was criticizing rural doctors for their poor practice because of the high admission rates in their hospitals. To give him credit, the specialist accepted the invitation of the rural practitioner and went to his town. The rural practitioner gave him the example of a child aged 10, at 11 o'clock at night developing acute asthma. The family lives on the dairy farm about an hour out of town so the child is brought in. What happens in that town is nebulizer treatment and so on, and then the child is admitted to the hospital and is kept overnight, in a stable atmosphere, observed by the nursing staff. This is beneficial to the parents who then can calm down, go back to the farm, get a few hours' sleep before they have to get up in the morning and milk the cows. It means the doctor can go back to bed at that time. In that community the doctor was on-call for 24 hours a day for a whole week at a time, and that certainly seemed like optimal care in that setting and what might be termed best practice in that context. The specialist looked into the distance and asked: 'Well, couldn't the child stay in a house in the town?' Of course he'd missed the point that the hospital is the 'house in the town', so I guess

I'm saying in different ways some of what's been said about locally developed mechanisms of care actually work better in that local setting; it's very much context-determined.

I wanted to pick up a bit about the after-hours and sustainability issues. Richard Hays and I were involved in a study, a number of years ago now, in Australia, looking at sustainable general practice in rural and remote communities.[157] We looked at 22 case studies in different remote communities – some were doing well and some weren't doing very well at all – and we looked to identify what the common themes were in sustainability. In the ones that were doing best, one of the things was active community participation in running the local health service, so there was some community representative organization, whether it was a hospital board or the municipality. Of course it varies in Australia from state to state, but that was a common theme. Another was the actual expectations of the doctor, so the worst stories that we could probably all tell around the table are examples where there's a mismatch of expectation between the community, what they expect in terms of medical services, and the doctor in what they are prepared to provide. It works best when there's an explicit agreement between the doctor and the community as to how long the doctor's going to stay in the community, the range of services provided, which addresses the issue that everyone wants to have their babies and have all kinds of surgery done in their local hospital and so on. That's not necessarily realistic, achievable, or advisable, not necessarily because of the doctor but because of nursing staff and facilities and resources and those sorts of things. Negotiating the range of services and the availability arrangements is very important. The ideal is in a one-doctor town, the solo practitioner being able to be off-call and at home and know that she won't be called. This can only happen if there is a safety net and the community knows the after-hours arrangements. We found in different communities that it might be networking between communities, so one doctor covers several communities after hours and weekends and so on; it might be nurses or nurse-practitioners taking a first line call, or in Australia it might be the Royal Flying Doctor Service, but I think that the key is actually having a system that people know and that they can rely on *and* trust. Coming back to the theme that Jim Douglas started; this may well be a situation where the way to deal with the situation that you've talked about is actually to learn from the rural setting and put in place new mechanisms or different approaches that have

---

[157] Monash University Centre for Rural Health, University of Queensland Northern Queensland Clinical School, Flinders University Rural & Remote Health Unit (1998).

actually been developed in the more isolated areas because they have no choice, like Fort William, but equally would work for the small village near Exeter – so a local network, not a national phone line and all the rest of that.

Pereira Gray: If we can, we should continue on national and international organizations and networks and communications.

Hays: A few years ago I was at a dinner party and the phone of the woman sitting opposite me rang; she was the person in North Queensland – a geographic area four times the size of the UK with a population of 700,000 – with the power to organize retrievals, and somehow a call had been escalated to her about a six-year-old boy whose mother had forgotten to take a Ventolin puffer home. It was going to be a cold night and they were worried about his asthma as he lived in a remote community in a valley 50 miles away, no air strip, dirt roads, they didn't have a car; there was a GP 30 miles away, half-way in between, but there was no mention of contacting the GP. She authorized a helicopter to fly a retrieval team, including a nurse and an ICU registrar, to lift this boy out of this valley on a winch to come into hospital. It turned out that he was admitted to hospital, he didn't have an asthma attack at all and he went home in a taxi the next day. There was some discussion about why she did that. Why didn't she call the local GP? Why didn't she send out an ambulance or a paramedic with a Ventolin puffer and a peak-flow meter? Of course, the answer was, and I think this is the impact of medical and legal things on rural medicine, that she said: 'Once this call was escalated to me the stakes were high, and if something had happened to that child, I would have lost my career, I would have lost my job and the service would have been brought into disrepute.' I think that the central planners actually don't understand rural medicine and healthcare. They design big systems that work in a different way and I think, as much as medical and rural health organizations are very effective at some things, something we haven't done so well is putting these options on the table, 'How do you connect in with the local healthcare services?' to come up with a more sensible solution than that.

Douglas: Can I just go back to the Working Time Directive because I think it is important in the historical narrative because the Working Time Directive was started in the UK in the mid-1990s?[158] I would like to speak in praise of

---

[158] The Council Directive 93/104/EC of 23 November 1993 concerned 'certain aspects of the organization of working time' including working hours, rest periods, breaks, annual leave, and shift work. This was superseded by Directive 2003/88/EC of the European Parliament and of the Council of 4 November 2003, online at http://eur-lex.europa.eu/legal-content/EN/ALL/?uri=CELEX:32003L0088 (accessed 23 May 2016).

the directive, as one with an occupational health interest. In fact, two days ago I read an article in *Occupational Medicine* about the impact of circadian rhythms and the upset of circadian rhythms on shift work, and there's a very definite correlation between shift work and adverse health outcomes, some of whom end up with cancer, heart trouble, and all that stuff.[159] I've no doubt about that evidence. As the father of two medical children, I'm very pleased that they are subject to the Working Time Directive; one of them is in surgical training and one of them is doing psychiatric training. The discussion about Working Time Directive is very much about 'How can you train the surgeons for the future?' I think that is all possible with a bit of common sense in the education side. I think if we're going back to questions about endurance and sustainability, how do we have sustainability? If the doctors say that we've got to have rigid rules like the Working Time Directive, the difficulty is how they are actually implementing it. So it's Gordon's point here – you've got absolutely rigid structures that you can't change on the local level. If for instance a young doctor like David comes along and says: 'Actually, I'm OK with being on-call and I want to go and sit in this rural community, despite the Working Time Directive, that's my free choice. I've read Dr Douglas' evidence in the journal or whatever it is that says it's going to cause me cancer, but I'm okay with it', then that's fine. I think we've got to have enough flexibility so that people can make that choice. The difficulties of systems that are so rigid, it's back to the central rigid systems, that you can't make personal choice. We do have to make sure that rural doctors or rural nurses or whoever have a work–life balance that is going to be allowed to be in place in the demographics for at least 40 years, because our children are going to last until their 90s or 100s and they're going to have to continue working up until 65/70 or whatever, so they most definitely have got to have a long-term work–life balance. The Working Time Directive, the work–life balance, is an important issue; yes, it has done harm, but I think it is potentially going to do more good than harm in the long term, both to the doctors and to their patients.

The other point I wanted to make was about the needs of rural communities and so on, and the technical advances of medicine treating things like heart attacks, strokes, etc. I can remember in the early part of my career there was an evidence base for saying you should treat people with MIs (myocardial infarction) at

---

[159] Arendt (2010). See also video clips and an edited interview with Professor Josephine Arendt online at www.histmodbiomed.org/article/josephine-arendt (accessed 23 May 2016) and comments at a Witness Seminar on seasonal affective disorder (SAD): Overy and Tansey (eds) (2014).

home, it was better than putting them into an intensive care unit.[160] Well, how that has completely changed around and somebody with a heart attack has to get to a super-specialist centre where they get balloon angiography straight away, etc.; the same with cerebrovascular accident, etc.; the same with people with major comas. No doubt we can't neglect that evidence and discriminate against rural people and say you can't get access to those treatments, but also we can do better in rural communities about care of the frail elderly, about the care of babies and children, and so on, that people don't necessarily need huge hi-tech care, they need common sense generalism on the ground. To me, it is all about trying to be flexible, it's all about trying to get the most appropriate care for the most appropriate illness, the most appropriate situation, flexibility and common sense, probably empowering the local community and the local professionals on the ground. It's the rigid things that get in the way; it's the rigid things that say: 'You can't do that because of whatever, whatever', and then it doesn't happen and nobody wins. So we've got to try to start empowering the professionals and the communities on the ground.

Sarah Strasser: I was thinking about the flexibility. The problem was, though, Jim, that if you had a bad night on-call you could cancel the following morning clinic and everyone would understand and you would be told, if you were a patient, that the doctor was on-call. That was a long time ago, but we went from being that flexible to being a bit more rigid to then having enforced rigidness. The other thing I just wanted to raise following on from Richard's comments reminded me that actually many of the practices that I had anything to do with were actually dispensing practices and that's also gone by the by.

Baird: We were asked about networking and I think it's about mutual understanding. I have to apologize about another anecdote but it is about dislocation of the shoulder. We had a dislocated shoulder in casualty and we'd just had an edict from the orthopaedic surgeons that we should not reduce dislocated shoulders in our department; they should all be sent to Dumfries, 75 miles away. Now this is fairly typical of the didactic approach, at a number of levels and it's like peeling an onion, you get these regionally, you get them supra-regionally, and you get them nationally, and I think we've got to avoid that. In order to resolve it, I phoned up, and there is a God because it was the

---

[160] Mather *et al.* (1976). Professor Sir Denis Pereira Gray wrote: 'This was a controlled trial in the South West of England. It showed little difference between treatment for adults with heart attacks with home treatment and the new coronary care units in hospital. For men over 60, it was statistically significantly safer to be treated by the GP at home.' Letter to Ms Caroline Overy, 19 August 2016.

orthopaedic surgeon who'd produced the diktat, and I said: 'I've three options here: I can send him through to Dumfries, which he refuses; I can do it in the department with an anaesthetist and reduce it under proper analgesia; or I can offer that I'll take him out to the car park and reduce it as a general practitioner'. He said, 'You're being stupid'. Now I guess it's easy to resolve it at that level at that time, but it should not have happened and the person who was being stupid about the patient was not, I think, me. I have to beat a drum here, but there is a disconnect and a lack of networking sometimes and mutual understanding even within regions. Actually, what do our College, our politicians, and the BMA do to keep us in the picture? Dispensing is a current issue and a lifeline for rural practices as well as an excellent service for patients. The BMA's doing little about it. The issue of funding temporary residents is another issue the BMA are doing little about even though the funding hasn't increased. Despite being a Fellow of the College I have not ever, in 30 years, been to a local faculty meeting, which is 85 miles and two-and-a-half hours away. I think networking and getting mutual understanding is important but we're not going to do it without some mutual movement, and I guess the challenge for the future is how we create that network because I think, frankly, it simply doesn't exist. Certainly since the 1990 contract, it's all been centrally imposed and since then things went downhill badly and have got progressively worse in terms of people understanding what our issues and problems are.

Tansey: For the record, could I just ask what happened to the patient? What did you do?

Baird: He got home in about 15 minutes.

Pereira Gray: Nice ending.

Cox: It would be remiss not to include the systematic under-funding of rural healthcare, particularly in England, and draw attention to the Jarman index, which was an urban-based index using urban-based criteria, including things like ethnic mix that didn't apply to rural practice.[161] Since then, the trick that's disadvantaged rural funding streams has been using age-adjusted morbidity data rather than crude morbidity data and not taking into account the older rural population. I referred to Sheena Asthana from Exeter who has shown that there's been systematic under-funding of rural healthcare.[162] That doesn't take

---

[161] The Jarman index was developed in the 1980s, combining GP workload with census variables to identify underprivileged areas: Jarman (1983).

[162] See, for example, Asthana, Halliday, and Gibson (2009).

into account the indirect costs – that's the opportunity costs for patients, their families, their employers – of people travelling to and from healthcare. I don't need to labour that or discuss it but that's for the record really.

Baird: Those economies of scale.

Pereira Gray: The next bit is to discuss education, and this has been a very interesting story, because when I first went into general practice there was a worldwide crisis of recruitment to rural practice. We have seen a remarkable development of a number of very innovative programmes and we're pretty fortunate here, around this table, to have two or three of those well represented. We've got to cover what it is the students need, what is the international training, what lessons can we learn, what is the academic programme, and what can the professional bodies do.

Roger Strasser: It started, I think, in the 1970s because there was such a shortage of rural doctors. Governments and medical schools came upon the idea that if the students spent some time in rural practice then some of them might like it and come back and then become rural practitioners, and it started just as a good idea.[163] Now, decades later, there's a lot of research that shows that that's actually true.[164] Subsequently the research has shown that there's a specific range of knowledge and skills that rural practitioners require, which has led to the inclusion of curriculum content around rural health and rural practice within many medical education programmes. In fact, just picking up on the workforce imperative for a moment, the research shows very clearly that the three factors most strongly associated with going into rural practice after education and training are, first of all a rural upbringing, that's having grown up in a rural area, that's the first factor; the second factor is positive – and I emphasize the word positive – clinical and educational experiences in the rural setting as part of undergraduate education; and then thirdly, at the postgraduate level targeted training that prepares the trainees with the skills they need to be rural practitioners. Those are the three factors that come together to be the main success factors for recruitment into rural practice after education and training.[165]

---

[163] Professor Roger Strasser added: 'For example, in 1971 the Minnesota Legislature threatened to cut funding to the University unless the School produced more rural doctors. This was the trigger for the Rural Physicians Associates Program initiated in Minnesota by Jack Verby.' See Verby (1988).

[164] See, for example, Wilkinson *et al.* (2003); Curran and Rourke (2004).

[165] See, for example, Strasser *et al.* (2016); Strasser and Neusy (2010).

But just coming back to the story about rural-based medical education, the idea was that if students tried rural practice they might like it, then found that there's actually a defined knowledge and skill set, and then as the evidence came through it became clear that the rural setting is actually a great place to learn clinical medicine for everybody. The students have much more patient contact, they have exposure to a wide range of clinical problems and common clinical problems, they get to develop their clinical and procedural skills, and now the evidence shows that students particularly having a prolonged learning experience in the rural practice and rural community setting actually develop a higher level of knowledge and skills and clinical confidence and competence than students who do the standard teaching hospital rotations, the block rotations in learning their core clinical medicine. There could be an argument that all medical students should have at least some rural clinical experience.[166] Certainly that's provided the basis for the development of rural-based medical schools and schools that have a specific mission or mandate focused on graduating doctors for rural practice. Of course, Richard Hays had the lead role with the James Cook University in Australia and Eldryd Parry at Ilorin in Nigeria and other places. I think one of the key aspects of all of these is the learning in the community that is sometimes described as community-based medical education or learning in context, so the students and the residents are learning in the community clinical setting. To understand how much that is a special feature of rural-based medical education, it's important to contrast that with, what for the best part of the twentieth century was, and maybe still is, the standard model of medical education where the clinical education takes place in the teaching hospital, which is a large acute urban centre. Certainly in the latter part of the twentieth century with increasing specialization, sub-specialization, technology in medicine, people have to be very sick, have a very rare condition, or require high technology intervention to actually become a patient in a teaching hospital.[167] They are in and out very quickly, so from a medical student's point of view, in that setting, you have to be quick to catch the patients to learn from them. Second, it's a very distorted clinical experience because the mix of patient problems in the teaching hospital setting is very far removed from the common clinical problems in the community. So community-based medical education, with students, certainly in general practice, but also in other health service settings – mental health services, long-term care facilities,

---

[166] See Worley *et al.* (2000).

[167] See Green *et al.* (2001).

the smaller community hospitals, and so on – has developed as part of rural-based medical education. This has now become a theme in broader medical education, and medical educators more generally are looking at community-based medical education as they are starting to realize the limitations of purely learning clinical medicine in the teaching hospital setting.

Hays: To add to that, I think in looking at what had to happen in James Cook University School of Medicine that has now graduated five groups,[168] I'll call it educational evidence for want of a better term, because there was a whole movement in Australia trying to examine how we could maximize the recruitment of rural doctors, and there's a complex package of all sorts of things at all levels but at James Cook we looked very hard at trying to skew admissions. We were getting 12 applicants for every place so why don't we choose the students who we thought were going to have the best chance of working in non-metropolitan, rural, and regional communities? It had to be politically broader than simply rural and remote, although it included that.[169] We actually built in a loading for going to certain rural schools; there are systems to do this and this has survived legal challenge, because it was challenged legally by somebody who was brought up in rural Iran and somehow felt aggrieved that we had left him out and we'd gone through three years of court work. We then looked at ruralizing the curriculum so that as much as possible teaching and assessment were contextualized in rural community stuff. One of my great colleagues, Craig Veitch, who has got connections with Inverness and the Remote and Rural Areas Resource Initiative (RARARI) as well, loves to say: 'If you've met one rural community, you've met one rural community.'[170] He's not the only person to have said that, of course, but you know, this was very strong for us, that if you accept that rural healthcare was so much about the community, the services and resources around it, the context, then to teach and assess in rural and regional context was essential. This created problems for us, because we had to write all of our own new curriculum materials and all our own assessment items. We discovered in joining an assessment consortium later – I'm currently the chair of the Ideal Consortium, which has got 36 members around the world – that James Cook couldn't get any assessment items from us

---

[168] See page 38 for a later review.

[169] Hays and Bower (2001).

[170] Professor Craig Veitch held the Chair of Rural Health at James Cook University from 2000. In 2007 he was appointed Professor of Community Based Health Care at the University of Sydney. For RARARI, see note 122.

because none of them were rural.[171] The third thing is we recruited as faculty very deliberately those who had been, or still at least were, positive promoters of rural medicine across specialties. What I'm saying is it's not just rural family practice or rural procedural medicine, but you had to get obstetricians and surgeons and physicians, the orthopod, who knew what it was like to be on the other end of the phone; we'd be getting people who knew what it was like to be out there and would be actively supportive. The curriculum model is that students all spend a minimum of 20 weeks in rural communities scattered over the six years of the course (it's a six-year course theme), but if they were interested, they could spend 100 weeks, which is a significant proportion of the course. Now, there are other schools with different models, and Roger Strasser's is one.[172] It's taken the one-year immersion model and adapted that to the Canadian system, another way of doing it, but in the evaluations the students at James Cook say that the best learning experience of the entire six years is what we call the 'rural internship', an eight-week block in their final year, just before graduation, where they are put in a rural hospital as apprentices and allowed to do all sorts of things – take calls, they are part of the system – and we had to do this against an edict from Queensland Health, who said this was illegal. So we approached rural doctors and said 'Queensland Health says it's illegal to involve students at this level of care, it breaks the rules, how about it?' Everybody said 'yes', because they saw just how sensible it was and what a role model. When it comes to the evaluations, four years in a row, it's rated the most valuable experience. Why? Because they were given some responsibility, they were given a broad range of exposure, they had been equipped with all the stuff about how to be there and do it and they'd been out there; they had rural e-mentors and rural face-to-face mentors. It's been quite interesting to see this construction of rural medical education based on what I am calling loosely the evidence.[173] There are evidence-based medicine (EBM) people who would probably criticize and you can talk about the four levels of evidence, but I'm not talking about that, it's about what emerges from the literature where sometimes it's just the

---

[171] Professor Richard Hays explained: 'Most assessment is context free, on the grounds that the context potentially clouds thinking and should not influence the correct answer. However, in rural medical education, context is regarded as important because sometimes different decisions are needed. Some of this is discussed in the following three papers: Smith and Hays (2004); Hays (2003a and 2003b).' Email to Ms Caroline Overy, 12 July 2016.

[172] See, for example, Strasser and Strasser (2007); Strasser *et al.* (2009). For a history of the Northern Ontario School of Medicine, see Tesson *et al.* (eds) (2009).

[173] See, for example, Sen Gupta *et al.* (2008).

experience, rather than a randomized controlled trial, which you can't do in education really. It's interesting to see that there are now several schools in the world that have taken similar approaches to try to build in what we know works and I think that, for me, as an educator, has been a fascinating experience.

Douglas: If we could just go over the historical thread of undergraduate training in general practice in the UK. It probably started in the first chair of general practice in the UK which was the University of Edinburgh, I think, in about 1963.[174] Then subsequently the other universities in Scotland, I believe in Glasgow, established departments of general practice and sent people, as part of their blocks, to remote and rural communities within Scotland, because of teaching capacity. So, for instance, the University of Aberdeen had an educational capacity problem, therefore, they sent their students up to the Islands of Orkney, etc. to gain experience in general practice. We have undergraduates in my practice and there's a very important function that general practice has in the whole undergraduate curriculum, and that's the one-to-one relationship that we have with the student when we've got them in our practice. Often, that's the first time in the whole of their undergraduate career that they've actually had one person looking at them, forming a relationship with them and observing them, even if it's just six to eight weeks. The rest of the time they can maybe pop in and pop out of a hospital ward or an outpatient department or whatever, and nobody sits and looks at them, so it's a very important function that general practice has in the whole system of undergraduate training that a proper personality assessment, educational assessment, communication skills assessment can be made. I think there's an important role for rural general practice teaching – we can explain the generality of things and we can explain generalism. There's a very important theme that, again, general practice has an important responsibility within the whole of medical education of treating, communication skills, of detailed assessment of the student, and I think that that is even better in the remote and rural context.

Roger Strasser: I'd just like to pick up on that theme. First of all to echo what you were saying I think there's quite a lot of evidence now that supports what you're saying. I recall some educators in Australia, probably about 20 years ago, did some research looking at rural general practitioners and their teaching of students and trainees in the rural setting. The heading of one of the articles they published said rural practitioners are 'naturally effective teachers' and

---

[174] Professor Richard Scott (*c.*1914–1983) was appointed to the newly established James Mackenzie Chair of General Practice at Edinburgh University in 1963: Anon (1984).

they demonstrated what they meant by that.[175] Certainly that's something that I've observed over the years that, not just rural general practice but all general practitioners, if they're good doctors, they've developed a whole lot of skills through their interactions with patients which are transferable into the teaching situation with individual students or groups. There's a close parallel process between the patient/doctor relationship and the learner/teacher relationship. The thing is that often the GPs don't see themselves as teachers because they've come from a medical school where their experience of medical education was lectures and ward rounds. They know that they're no good at lectures and they don't do teaching ward rounds, so they don't see themselves as teachers. So one of the challenges is to help them to recognize the skills that they have, that they've developed through their patient interactions and have confidence in themselves as teachers. That brings me back to the theme, I said that the evidence shows there's positive clinical and educational experience at the undergraduate level. Jim Douglas talked about what motivated sending the students into the rural general practice setting was capacity concerns. Unfortunately, I've seen this happen too often in many parts of the world where the teaching hospital's getting overcrowded and so the decision is taken to send the students out to a rural setting – it could be a rural hospital or a rural general practice – and the mindset is that it's getting the students out from underfoot and so there's a negative spin to this and so the students go because they're told they have to. They go seeing this is a bad thing, more or less by definition; as they expected, they have a bad experience and so it adds to the negativism around rural practice. This all derives from, I guess in the big picture as we heard earlier, the assumption in the large urban areas that anything that happens outside the city is, by definition, second class or of a lesser standard. Then the predominance of specialists and sub-specialists and, of course, it's the specialists and sub-specialists that dominate the teaching hospital. Their standing assumption is that, well, you know, if you're not good enough to become a specialist in a teaching hospital then maybe you can be a specialist in another hospital, and if you can't be a specialist in another hospital maybe you can be a GP, and the ultimate default is to become a rural general practitioner. The students pick up these negative assumptions and perceptions, so they go out to the rural setting with a negative mindset. For some of them, of course, it's such a good experience that that's turned around, but for others it's self-fulfilling. The fact that often, without some encouragement, the rural GPs are so self-effacing also tends to add to this negativism. A key, really, is to ensure that it's set up in a

---

[175] Miflin and Price (1993).

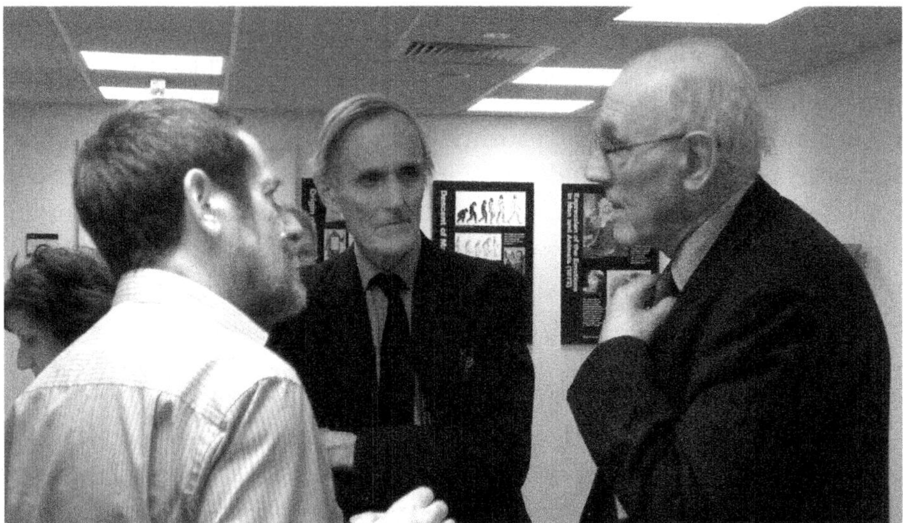

Figure 36: Professor Roger Strasser, Professor Sir Eldryd Parry
and Professor Sir Denis Pereira Gray

way that is seen as important and valuable and positive for the students and then that's reinforced, not only in terms of the GP but the whole – the health team and the wider community as was mentioned earlier. I'd like to ask Eldryd Parry to say a few words about his experiences in establishing community-based medical education.

Professor Sir Eldryd Parry: Perhaps I may say first of all that in this company my credibility must be that I am the child of two general practitioners and my sister had a chair of primary care in the University of Iowa. I've been a physician, trained at the Hammersmith and at the National Heart Hospital by Paul Wood, who was the leading cardiologist,[176] and that was going to be my line until I was seconded from the Hammersmith to Ibadan University College Hospital in Nigeria. We went six days after we married and that altered the course of my life and my wife's life. We spent two and a half years there, when Hammersmith had said only one, and we had hoped to return to do research but there was no funding. I was invited to Ethiopia at the beginning of the medical school and saw the first graduates through and then I was invited to set up a department of medicine in northern Nigeria, in Zaria, where we had substantial emphasis

---

[176] Dr Paul Hamilton Wood (1907–1962) was a cardiologist at British Postgraduate Medical School at Hammersmith Hospital from 1935 to 1948; he was Director of the Institute of Cardiology at the National Heart Hospital, and cardiologist to the Brompton Hospital, London, until his death in 1962. See Campbell (1962).

upon rural work because our concept of medicine was that it wasn't something that only happened in a hospital. As Professor of Medicine I was to take my students into the field every Friday afternoon. From there I was invited to set up a new medical school in Nigeria by Professor Oladipo Akinkugbe, who was one of Nigeria's most esteemed academics and we wanted to do something radical for the needs of the country, so we did.[177] We took the students to live with us in the community on day one of year one and that was quite acceptable to Tamas Fulop, who was head of the WHO education group then. The community-orientated group of medical schools was started in 1979 and I was a founder member of that.[178] Unfortunately it got hijacked by the northern problem-based established schools; McMaster[179] and Maastricht moved in with the armoury and the money and the numbers so that those of us who were rural pioneers or were doing unusual things got outnumbered, and our group became dominated by problem-based learning, and people pretended that there was community orientation because students went into homes rather than spending their whole time in the hospital. After that I was invited to, I suppose the word would be, 'rescue' a medical school in Ghana where I was Dean at Kumasi for five years.[180] We then came home and on coming home I realized that our historic responsibilities for developing countries were being jettisoned rapidly in the UK in education and so, with some friends, we set up THET (Tropical Health & Education Trust), a charitable trust, and this is now a strong agency for establishing training links with counterparts in the poor world and that means in a few African countries.[181]

---

[177] Professor Oladipo Olujimi Akinkugbe (b. 1933) was a lecturer in the Department of Medicine at University of Ibadan, Nigeria from 1965; he became Professor of Medicine in 1968, and was Dean from 1970 to 1974. In 1975 he was appointed Vice-Chancellor of the new University of Ilorin, and in 1979 as Vice-Chancellor of Ahmadu Bello University, Zaria, Nigeria, where he stayed for only one year. See his autobiography: Akinkugbe (2010).

[178] See Schmidt *et al.* (1991).

[179] McMaster Medical School developed a course for self-directed, problem-based learning with continuous assessment; see Spaulding (1991).

[180] Professor Sir Eldryd Parry was Dean and Professor of Medicine at the Kwame Nkrumah University of Science and Technology, Kumasi, Ghana, from 1980 to 1985.

[181] Professor Sir Eldryd Parry established THET (Tropical Health & Education Trust) in 1988, a charity to support health workers, and establish health partnerships, in low- and middle-income countries in Africa, Asia, and the Middle East; he chaired the organization from its beginning until 2007. See the website at www.thet.org/ (accessed 25 May 2016). An interview with Professor Parry was conducted by Professor Tilli Tansey in July 2016 and is available on our website at www.histmodbiomed.org/.

To go back to what you were saying, you mentioned a health team and teaching, you talked about people being reluctant to learn as teachers. One of the great lessons I have learned is that, where a health team is being taught in a school of health sciences, of which a medical school is part, for that health team to work in the community together, naturally there's leadership, usually from a doctor, although it may not be, and they learn: (a) to work to each other; and (b) to encourage and help each other. It isn't enforced, you have to learn how to teach but effectively they know that's how they're going to work for the rest of their lives and, therefore, they begin to relate to each other and they begin to learn how to communicate and to teach each other. I shall soon be in such a place, working with a man who pioneered that 'team training', as he calls it, in southern Ethiopia.

One word about James Cook and the selection of students: we did this in northern Nigeria in the 1960s. There was a great push from the south, where there was an excess of qualified students who couldn't get into the few elite medical schools to come to the north. Our medical school was set up in the north to provide doctors from the north so we had a discriminating admissions policy and I knew the sub-tribal map of northern Nigeria better than my colleagues. There was a very good colonial office map, which showed the smaller tribal areas and we looked at the address of where the boys came from (there were very few girls at that stage) and actually discriminated in their favour. The astonishing thing about this was if we brought them on, frequently they did far better, and to extrapolate from that to the Ilorin experience, which I'll come on to in a moment,[182] we took the cast-offs from Ibadan, Lagos, and the big centres, and because we gave them an exciting education, rather than a didactic one, when they went to Ibadan to do their clinicals they came top, which was very surprising because actually we'd taken them through an education where problems were important. I wouldn't say it was fully problem-based, because that leads me to another point. My philosophy of education is not to be doctrinarian and say 'This will be problem-based', but to say 'Given our current circumstances, what is the best way that this group of students at this time in their course can reach the educational goals?', or the competencies, however you wish to express them, and that may be problem-based. It may be practical skills sitting in a casualty department, I don't know, but I think that's a very important thing and unfortunately, the community-based, the international rural medicine (which was what our group was) became a problem-based manqué group, because problem-based learning became a doctrine rather than a tool; to me problem-based learning is a tool, no more.

---

[182] See the comments on Ilorin by Professor John Hamilton on pages 22 and 45.

To go on a little bit, it's easy in a poor country if you're told to be radical to be radical because there are fewer committees and councils and things like that, and you just get on and do it. Students like that and like to be part of it. One thing you were saying about students feeling this was a second best; if they were told when they come into the schools that the whole philosophy of the school is towards this then they realize what they're doing is part of the philosophy of the school. If they see their own ideal future is being a super-specialist in a hospital then they've probably gone to the wrong medical school. But I think it's very important for the philosophy to be understood and to be embraced. Our students were proud. Let me give you another illustration of this. We were desperately short of teachers of physiology in Ghana and yet we had some very bright fifth-year students, and I said: 'I don't want them to learn classic physiology, I want them to learn clinical physiology, at the bedside if possible.' So, I took a group of seven of the best, who were volunteers, to patients illustrating problems of fluids. It's no problem finding an oedematous patient; it's no problem to find someone with diarrhoea who was dehydrated; we looked at the physical signs and we looked at what the issues were and discussed them. The second-year students were taught by our fifth-year that day. What did the second-year students say? 'What a fantastic medical school we're in if the fifth-year students are so good!' So, from having our backs to the wall with no teachers, they believed they were in the best place. And what did it do to the confidence of our students? One gave a paper at the World Congress of Tropical Medicine in Calgary in 1984 on this very issue and he was acclaimed, which is again quite a lesson.[183] A senior student or junior intern can be a useful resource where people are a problem. I would like to go on but I don't want to interfere with the general theme of general practice, but I think these are important and interesting.

McNicol: Two things. I've been involved with students for 35 years, in fact the first student I ever taught as a GP registrar was the senior lecturer in general practice at Glasgow University, who had no general practice experience whatsoever. He was a bit mortified the next year when, as a visiting senior lecturer in general practice, he came out to Newfoundland where I was a registrar in general practice; when he saw me there he said, 'Oh dear!' But education

---

[183] Jacob Plange-Rhule graduated from the School of Medical Sciences of the Kwame Nkrumah University of Science and Technology in 1984. He became Consultant Physician in Komfo Anokye Teaching Hospital where he set up the Hypertension and Renal Clinic, and was Head of the Department of Physiology of the School of Medical Sciences, Kumasi. He is now the Rector of the Ghana College of Physicians and Surgeons (https://gcps.edu.gh/?page_id=2181 accessed 16 November 2016).

has changed tremendously. In the 1970s, it was 'follow the GP round' and do whatever – they usually came with guitars over their shoulder, a list of phone numbers of girlfriends to phone, and disappeared for days on end. There is now a much more structured list of tasks to do. The Aberdeen students that I've had until my retirement had very much work to do in the eight weeks, so things have changed tremendously there. The most interesting education that I've done was this project with Middlebury College in Vermont where we had a liberal arts college with straight-A students heading for medicine, and the Professor of Anthropology, David Napier, had done some research – 35 per cent of American medical students by the time they got to third year in medicine decided they didn't want to do medicine and only 65 per cent did.[184] By that stage they were between $250,000 and $300,0000 in debt and all they could do to pay that debt off was to keep going in medicine and become high-volume ENT surgeons, dermatologists, whatever. The basis of what we were trying to do in Middlebury was get these bright students who were being told: 'You're getting straight-As, so be a doctor, be a lawyer, that's where the money is', to actually sample general practice, rural practice and, basically, medicine. They came over and spent a month living with us and doing things, and some of them were absolutely fired up and decided this was what they wanted to do and, in fact, three or four of them already are running departments of rural medicine in the US. One of the most successful ones was a girl who came and wanted to be a model at the Sorbonne – she had no interest in people; in Scotland, she never asked a question in a month and I wrote in her summation: 'This girl should not be practising medicine.' Middlebury were furious: 'What right have you got to tell us about these straight-A students?' But then 9/11 came along and they changed their attitude a bit. She wrote to me, and I saw her some time later, and she said: 'I've decided to become a chiropractor and I'm so glad I'm not doing medicine.' There is a scope in medical education at a stage – in the British system it would be quite hard to know when – to actually expose pre-medical people to medicine just to make sure they want to do it, because we do see some people in fifth-year medicine and you think: 'Why are you here?' That's very sad for everybody.

Baird: We were talking about recruitment problems in the 1970s. In 1984 I advertised for a partner in Galloway and there were 80 applicants. In the Lake District a practice advertisement got 240 applicants. With the work I had for

---

[184] See Flaherty (1998).

writing to 80 applicants I was amused to find out that they (in the Lake District) omitted in the advertisement to say it was part-time and had to write 240 letters and re-advertise asking if the doctors were still interested. Recruitment difficulties in rural practice are relatively recent, within the last 20 years.[185] My assessment of why this has happened – and we wrote about it in the *Occasional Paper* – is about balancing proactive and reactive care, and I think the 1990s introduced a proactive element to practice, which is difficult to implement with people that you know very well and to appear to be didactic.[186] I think an unintended consequence of that was the relative devaluing of reactive care because you can't just add something in and not take something away if resource is finite. I think anticipatory care in terms of it is a fashion and in terms of funding is in the ascendancy. I think this devaluation has changed us from being patient-centred, which is sometimes described as the GP being social capital, which is a reactive and an exciting and involving thing, to a doctor-based or system-based model of health, which doesn't relate well to small communities and particularly when it's commodity-based as medicine has increasingly become. That's happened gradually over the last 20 years. The interesting thing is that in the 1990s I advertised again and the only applicant I got was an ex-registrar, so I think from what you're saying from Australia and from international commentary is borne out by personal experience. I guess we do have to change the value set between proactive and reactive care that politicians and managers have and, while I think training is important, I think infusing people with reactive and interventional and patient-centred care is important. David Hogg wants to be a rural GP. He can't decide where he's going to be at rural training; he's actually got an urban posting and he wants to be rural – that's a dismal reflection on the selection process. There are opportunities for five-year training in the Rural Fellowship Scheme, although the Rural Fellowship Scheme is quite small, but five-year training is an opportunity.[187] Undergraduate teaching is certainly the key, and many medical schools are now doing this and we get good feedback, and I think this has to be developed in community hospitals. Moving towards clearer pathways for tertiary care is also important.

Douglas: Could I start drawing out some of the themes about the UK versus the international dimension? I think, as I've indicated, probably in the UK, certainly in Scotland, we've been doing remote and rural healthcare for many years and

---

[185] See also the comments by James Douglas and recruitment problems on page 34.

[186] Gillies, Baird, and Gillies (1995).

[187] For the one-year Rural Fellowship Scheme in Scotland, see MacVicar, Clarke, and Hogg (2016).

sending students out into practices, and so on. I think the great thing that the international community has given us, in other words what Roger Strasser, Richard Hays, the people in America, and all the other parts of the world, because of their different health systems and, to take the Australian example, because they had the political problem to solve and they got the politicians involved – there were votes in rural areas and something had to be done about the rural areas. In the UK, I think we've gained a great deal in that you formalized it for us and you established departments of rural health, departments of rural medicine, and so on, and although we were doing it, the contribution that the international dimension has given to us in the UK is to say that there is a specialty. Your problems of remote and rural-ness are probably 'worse' than ours – you've got the bush and you've got indigenous people/medicine, all these sorts of things – so, in many ways, you've got more challenging remote and rural issues, but I think the circle has now begun to be squared. The fact that you've highlighted it, what did happen, we went through a period in the UK where when the problems started coming in remote and rural healthcare and our politicians in Scotland or wherever were getting a bit twitched up that they were going to lose votes: 'Somebody else in the world must know the solution to this problem, go and find out what the Australians have done, go and find out what the Norwegians have done or whatever.' The fact we're probably doing it already but the international community has done us a big service in the UK, certainly from the Scottish perspective, in defining the specialty and taking it forward for us. Within the UK we've got to build on that, and the whole business about professional identity and self-belief of remote and rural practitioners; I think that's a very important thing for sustainability.

Sustainability of rural communities is that the people within that community are feeling comfortable – that they can have babies, they can have heart attacks, and all the rest of it, they're going to be safe in that community, their children are going to be educated, etc. But part of the sustainability is also that the rural practitioner is comfortable living within that community, they're comfortable in their skin, and they're comfortable living within the goldfish bowl. Preparing them for that eventuality is an important thing and that's one of the things that we have been trying to do, certainly in Scotland with our GP Rural Fellowship, which is a postgraduate fellowship. Once people have done their vocational training in general practice, they are allowed to practise anywhere in the UK, so although we train people in the rural context they should, at the end of the day, be able to work in Birmingham as well as in Orkney. Once they've got that bit of paper, we then give them another year's experience, a safe experience in general practice, and begin to try to address some of the issues like professional isolation, social isolation, and consider some of the issues about: 'How do you like living in the middle of a goldfish bowl and everybody knowing your business?' Hopefully then people at the end of that year can then make informed choices about whether they want to live in a rural community or not. A lot of that thinking has come from Australia and Canada and so on, and within the UK context I would like to thank our colonial colleagues for allowing us to take some of that thinking a bit further forward.

Hays: I just want to talk about comparing England in particular to the Australian experience. In Australia there was the Government push as you say. There was money available; people like Roger and I were given the authority to go and do interesting things. In my case I benefited from living 1,000 miles by road from my metropolitan employer. They were interested to know what I was doing and I was far more in touch with the local community, because I'd been to school there and I'd worked there for 20 years, 15 years as a clinician. I was daring to be different and able to be different and get away with it, and I think that it actually came as quite a surprise to my employer that, what I think they started as a soft political option, became not just one of the largest groups of the medical school, but in fact we were the largest-ranked getter and publishers of academic research in that medical school, which is a very large medical school.[188] We were able to be different and innovative, and I think Australia probably has a slightly more 'can do' attitude than England – I'm sorry Jim, I can only talk about England, not the rest of the UK. But, I found coming to Keele, where, for a start, there were then two GPs on the medical school's council, so of the 32 heads of medical school, two were GPs. In Australia nine of the 19 are GPs, I'm told, the majority with a rural background. Now, at Keele, there's now only one GP on the medical school's council of 32 with a primary care background. The emphasis here is on elite, academic, biomedical, and extraordinarily narrow specialists, teaching research right from the very beginning. I did this as an exercise when I came here, I looked at the vision statements and mission statements of every medical school in the UK to find that most of them had one except they'd say 'If you come to us you'll be taught by Nobel prizewinners', which I think is probably a slight distortion of the truth. If you talk to students who apply to medical schools in the UK, as I have done, they're not thinking about rural practice, they're making choices based on the fact that students can

---

[188] James Cook University was founded in 1970 and the College of Medicine and Dentistry established in Townsville, Queensland, in 2000. See, for example, Hays (2001).

only apply for four medical schools and they may take the only one they get into, but they do things like looking at 'I want to be taught by the very best' and there is a perception that the very best occurs in a very small number of the medical schools.

It's interesting to talk to the people who apply for Keele as a new school. I went out and sat in the waiting room at admissions day; I was talking to these people. I got feedback on the web and somebody said: 'We're not too sure who this old guy was, we wondered if he was a mature-age applicant, we found out later he was the Dean', there's a quote on the web somewhere. I'd say: 'Why did you apply here and what was the reply?' I discovered there is a group of students who actually deliberately apply to new medical schools, in England. Why? Because they say they want to do something different. They want to get out of their comfort zone, they want to get away from the traditional view. I've tried to start conversations at Keele about: 'How are we going to attract more of these people, they're the ones I'd go for?' The worst medical students we found at Keele are those who wanted to get into a London medical school, applied for three London schools with Keele as a backup and sadly only got Keele and stupidly came. They hate it, because it's not what they wanted. But what I've discovered is the medical community around me actually aspires to the Oxbridge golden triangle model as well. They do not believe that they should stick their neck above the parapet. Stand out and try to say we're doing something better than the golden triangle because we're offering a better educational learning experience and a more diverse range. I actually think I'm leaving England at probably the wrong time because Keele is about to start what will effectively be a rural clinical school along the Welsh border and, of course, where the Welsh border is depends on which country you're in. We're in a narrow band here from Worcestershire and then into Montgomeryshire, and we're just negotiating building accommodation, providing travel grants, and we're recruiting a great network of practices. Now I'm leaving before this is finalized, but I think it will still be successful. This is not new for Scotland, but it's very new for England and the thought that students might deliberately want to turn their back on the academic centres of excellence to go to learn about real healthcare and real people is not popular. I think that it is organizations, and maybe people like those who are in this room, who have got to take up this fight to make this a viable alternative for applicants.[189]

Parry: Can I ask one question? Why are you building accommodation?

---

[189] See further comments by Professor Hays on Keele University Medical School on page 39.

Hays: We're not; we're getting a grant to work with a local community, a charity to adapt some accommodation that is currently vacant, to the student requirements. You want them to live with the real doctors?

Parry: No, I believe that once you've got a fixed centre you're bound by that centre, you're bound by that rural building. You can't be flexible.

Hays: Yes, but it's a two-and-a-half hour's drive from Keele, so we have to provide accommodation or they don't go.[190]

Parry: Well, there are other models where students have to find their own.

Hays: That is revolutionary for England.

Cox: There's a conceptual point here that's not unique to medicine, but it's certainly happening with rural healthcare and what we're talking about, which is whether we're talking about a problem or an asset, the deficit model or the asset model. It's interesting in European legislation, if you look at the definitions of the Uplands, the mountain regions of Europe, in European law they're described as less favoured areas, disadvantaged areas, severely disadvantaged areas, or natural handicap areas. It's all about problems and that culture leads to: 'We need subsidies, we need help, it's a problem; we can't cope.' On the other hand, you could look at the European upland-belt, the Lake District, the Scottish Highlands and say actually these are huge assets. Not only are they beautiful, they produce most of the country's water, they're potentially places for renewable energy, landscape, recreation, health, tourism, all the assets. What Roger Strasser and Richard Hays are talking about is using the assets of rural areas to bring students on, the time that rural doctors have, the skills that they have, the role models that they are, the confidence that they can build, the evidence that's emerging and the way that can help recruitment. In a sense, in the UK, we haven't reached that level of maturity yet and we're still using the deficit model, instead of saying: 'This is a huge asset, not only can some rural general practices offer a medical education that will compete with Oxford and Cambridge; actually you need this because in many ways it's better.'

Hogg: I'll just quickly make a couple of points about career guidance. I think that for myself and my colleagues, and I know for my friends who have been through medicine, it's a recurring theme that we feel there could be more career guidance, and for protecting the future of rural practice I think it's a particularly pertinent point. I'll split it into basic categories. There's formal

---

[190] Bartlett *et al.* (2011).

careers guidance, which you can find on websites, that's been formally delivered in a less interactive fashion. The reason I think that rural placements work particularly well for encouraging people into both general practice and rural practice is that it's informal and interactive. It's attractive for students going out with a GP in the car during house visits, over coffee, they get to see the whole work–life balance. I think it's that access to career guidance that's particularly strong in general practice, and again particularly rural practice. Splitting it more chronologically: careers guidance can happen pre-university and I think that there are some fantastic schemes already set up in the UK, in pockets of the UK, which address that. We need to recognize that one of the main challenges for pre-university career guidance is that it's very difficult for rural pupils to access the local GPs for work experience, because confidentiality is an even bigger issue. I don't know if there needs to be a more national solution or at least something led by some of the professional bodies like the GMC or the RCGP or medical schools. At university there is, certainly in terms of training, I completely agree with the idea that you see that continuity. My experience of undergraduate training is great, but you go into hospital, you spend a lot of time chasing consultants, it's relatively fractured, you have days in and days out doing different things, and you rarely have the opportunity to see patients during the natural history of their disease. But you do see that with your patients in general practice and that's a huge strength, one I think we ought to build on, particularly because the continuity is being quickly eradicated in hospitals, because of short bed stays – you just don't see that any more in the big centres. In terms of postgraduate career guidance, I think there's a big need for better guidance, partly to promote rural practice and also to make sure that people don't make the wrong decision. I think that's particularly important for general practice now that we have a run-through training programme that looks likely to be extended to five years; you can very quickly find yourself in a programme where it is defined from year one what you're going to be doing for the next three, possibly five, years.[191] For both these reasons if you want to do rural practice it would be nice to have large elements of that in your training and vice versa. Having said that, we still need to recognize the generic skills of general practice and medicine in general and

---

[191] Run-through training programmes provide specialty training following the two-year Foundation Programme undertaken after graduation. Dr David Hogg wrote: 'The GP training programme is presently [2016] 3–4 years. It was being extended to include an optional 4th year at the time of the seminar. There are ongoing efforts to extend the programme to 5 years but as yet this has not taken place.' Email to Ms Caroline Overy, 5 July 2016.

I wouldn't want to be negative about my more urban-based training, where a lot of core generic skills can certainly be picked up there first and expanded later on. However, the relative flexibility of run-through training, which has some advantages, needs to be recognized. Those are basically the points I was going to mention, particularly themes of MTAS (Medical Training Application Service) and MMC (Modernising Medical Careers)[192] making sure that there is flexible and accessible careers guidance. I think these are particularly strong factors for protecting rural practice in the future.

Sarah Strasser: What works in the most remote site will likely work elsewhere in the healthcare system, and I'd like to report that what works for remote general practice or rural general practice educational training is likely to actually improve medical educational training across the board and so we do need to, as Richard pointed out, get faculty who are onboard and supportive. I guess what I'm conscious of is that we haven't discussed gender and where the female practitioner comes in and where the female student comes in, and I do want to suggest that if we do get it right for women you'll get it right for everybody else as well.

Douglas: Picking up Sarah's point about gender at the moment – there's an important point, if we're talking about the history of medical education and the history of evidence-based medicine, about the context of evidence. We talk a lot in modern healthcare about the context of where a study has been conducted and the bit that's often missing out of this, when we're talking about the way the guidelines are applied or where the services are developed and the valuations and so on, often a research study may be done in a hospital context in a city but then applied unthinkingly into a rural area. There's an important point in evidence-based medicine that one of the boxes that everybody should have to tick – and it's a development of the rural-proofing idea that came out of John Wynn-Jones' history of rural health in Wales[193] – in the teaching of evidence, this in terms of teaching undergraduates medicine and rural health and so on, we've got to understand the context of that evidence. An example,

---

[192] The postgraduate training programme in the UK, MMC (Modernising Medical Careers), was introduced in 2005 to reform postgraduate medical education. See UK Health Departments (2004). MTAS (Medical Training Application Service) was set up by MMC in 2007 as an online service for selecting and allocating posts to junior doctors. The service was hugely criticized by the medical profession, which led to the Independent Taskforce of Enquiry (Tooke Report), which exposed the arrangements and led to the complete failure of the system: Tooke (2008).

[193] For rural proofing, see page 36.

which I often say when I'm talking about this with students, is that if you do a study in Aberdeen Maternity Hospital in which you say that there's a midwifery-led maternity unit right beside a consultant high-tech unit, and from your study you may say that the maternal mortality rates and perinatal mortality rates and outcomes in the midwifery-led unit are absolutely perfect and therefore we should go as a country completely over to midwifery-led care. Well, that's fine if next door or down the corridor is the consultant-led unit and the instant Caesarean section, but you can't then go and apply that evidence to Orkney or Shetland or the islands where a Caesarean section is maybe many hours away and that's all about the context of where evidence is derived from. That's an important thing that we have to get, certainly in undergraduate education, we have to understand the context. There's another thing that I want to develop, another geographical context. I think in the UK we have a lot of government attention, both north and south of the border, about so-called health inequalities. For example, if you live in a deprived part of Glasgow in, say, Easterhouse, your life expectancy as a male is something like 60, whereas across the golf course in Lenzie in the middle-class area, the life expectancy of males is about 80; the difference in life expectancy is the most extreme example of health inequalities. The governments within civil society and western society realize that that is wrong; there's a moral deficit in the way we organize our current society and therefore a lot is put into trying to address health inequalities.[194] I think there's a common bond that we should have in undergraduate medical education between people trying to solve the inner city problems and rural health problems. Richard Hays has said that he has found many inner city doctors just as isolated as, if not more isolated than, rural doctors, because of networks and so on. Often the debate in the state-funded system in Britain in the NHS swings in a pendulum between trying to do something politically about inequalities in the inner cities and then trying to keep the remote rural areas onboard. The answer, obviously, is that, in our perspective anyway, we mustn't fight these people, we certainly mustn't say that we've got more difficult problems than the inner city people, we're both working from the same problem; we're working from a geographical deficit or we've got a geographical problem to solve. Theirs is all about transient communities, immigrant communities, cultural disorder, etc.; ours is about political disharmony and political distance and so on. If we're thinking about where we are at the moment in remote and rural healthcare and where we're

---

[194] Strategies for reducing inequalities in health in England were addressed in the Marmot Review published in 2010: Marmot (2010).

going towards in the future, we've got to start thinking about the inequalities of gender and we've got to form strategic alliances with those people who are battling in the inner city areas of London and our 'enemy' (in inverted commas) is not probably the person in the leafy suburbs but our friends are the people working in the inner cities.

Roger Strasser: I'd certainly support the notion of strategic alliances, shall we say, but I think, picking up on the deficit/asset concept, over the years talking about professional identity and role models, one of the challenges that's been experienced by rural doctor organizations in different countries has been to get the balance right. On the one hand, particularly in the political arena, to thump the table and talk about the way in which rural doctors are disadvantaged and should have better support in one way or another from the system and from the Government and so on. On the other hand, if they paint too bleak a picture then no medical students and new graduates are going to want to come and join them in rural practice, so the importance of actually highlighting that most rural practitioners are enjoying being rural practitioners. What attracts them is the variety of practice, and the environment in the broader sense. Most rural doctors enjoy the outdoor activities and so on. They enjoy looking after people with all kinds of health problems, the continuity and the comprehensive nature of the practice, and also providing, in a sense, the care for all of the medical problems, the continuity of care, and the special relationship with the community.

We've had a few comments about career guidance, even before medical school, to educate and to encourage. One of the key issues is actually to present pictures like that book with the photographs of the solo practitioners and their stories, examples and images and models that are positive about rural practice because that's how we're going to attract new recruits.[195] Earlier I said that there were three factors strongly associated with going to rural practice;[196] the first one is a rural upbringing. That highlights the importance of actually promoting healthcare as a career option for students in high schools, even in primary schools, in rural areas because they don't necessarily think of it. In fact, in my experience in the early days with Monash Rural Health, the rural students who got into Monash University were the stubborn ones. They weren't going to let their careers teacher talk them out of becoming doctors. The careers

---

[195] See page 105 and note 143.

[196] See page 122.

teacher would say: 'Don't get ideas above yourself', which of course is part of this acceptance of what happens, the rural are second class and being a rural student you can't possibly expect to do as well. This, of course, then translates in the rural community as a collective inferiority complex. Career guidance, even before getting into university and medical school, is very important and again I'm reminded of John MacLeod, who was a crusader for rural medicine in general and one of his methods was in getting the pupils into practice and encouraging them to think about medicine and health.[197] I think that there are ways of doing that to get around the confidentiality and anonymity aspects and then creating that sense of a career pathway that starts before university and into medical school.[198]

I want to pick up on – and this ties in very much with the comment made by Eldryd Parry and a few others about the philosophy of the medical school – that I think that it is key that the whole school has a clear and well-stated mandate. In the Australian context, James Cook University stood out as being established with a mandate that was focused, as Richard said, on rural and remote and Aboriginal health. Similarly, where I am now in Canada, Northern Ontario School of Medicine, the school was established as a result of a strong community movement and was established with, what we describe as, a social accountability mandate – that's a commitment to be responsive to the needs of the people and the communities of Northern Ontario. In fact, in the world of medical education, the notion of a medical school having a social accountability mandate is gaining momentum. It was first described in the mid-1990s by the World Health Organization as the obligation that the school has to tailor its education, research, and service to the needs of the region or the community that it's there to serve.[199] There are a growing number of medical schools around the world that have been established with a social accountability mandate.[200] In fact, James Cook University and Northern Ontario School of Medicine are two of eight medical schools around the world that have formed what's called a Training for Health Equity network (THEnet), and we're working at developing an evaluation framework and a mechanism for better demonstrating

---

[197] For John MacLeod see page 35 and note 40, and pages 106–7.

[198] See earlier comments by Dr David Hogg on page 138.

[199] Boelen and Heck (1995); Boelen, Dharamsi, and Gibbs (2012); Boelen and Woollard (2009); Woollard (2006).

[200] See, for example, Strasser *et al.* (2009); Strasser (2016); Murray *et al.* (2012).

and documenting what we're doing and how we connect what we're doing to responding to the needs of the communities that we're there to serve.[201] I think that that's important because it creates a different definition of the very best. In a sense, rural medical education will have been successful when we have medical graduates out there who aspire to be the very best rural and remote medical practitioners, certainly see themselves as assets to the system, and are doing the research and providing the evidence to demonstrate how in their communities they're improving the whole system in ways that are transferable into larger, even into the urban, centres. I think that's a direction which we're looking to go and then providing role models for the students and the new graduates, which comes back to the ongoing relationship that learners particularly have with rural practitioners.

Hays: I want to bring up marketing to potential students because I've had a lot to do with this over the years and something that I think scares a lot of young people is the promotion of what I came to call the 'ten-foot-tall bullet-proof rural doctor'. In this room I'm aware we've got some outstanding long-term, life sentence-type rural doctors. You've loved it and you've done very well and that's fantastic, but I've got to tell you, in my experience in Australia, that is not the long-term career ambition of many young people. They see themselves as being able to move around and do different things, so at James Cook University in particular we actually talk about: 'We will train you and set you up to be confident and be able to do well in rural practice, but if you only want to give it three or five years, that's great, you'll actually be a far better urban practitioner if you finish.' I was involved in some research that shows quite clearly that a key time when people move out of rural practice is when their eldest child gets to secondary school, because there are concerns about sending kids away to boarding school and stuff like that, which may be more real in Australia than here.[202] There's very good evidence that rural practice is a fantastic opportunity for a few to several years and I think that if we have a population of rural doctors, who include some like you guys who are there for the long term, the senior mentors, but even with a whole lot of people who drop in and out for five or ten years you're going to have a very good workforce. It's very important for younger people to realize that there is life after rural medicine. People do extraordinarily well. I could write a book about people

---

[201] See the Training for Health Equity Network website at http://thenetcommunity.org/ (visited 28 June 2016). For an evaluation of the framework see Ross *et al.* (2014).

[202] Hays *et al.* (1997).

who were in rural practice and are now doing fantastic things. A period in rural medicine actually sets you up to be an excellent practitioner, probably quite academically attuned, because you have to observe and record and interact with what's going on locally. Many academics are rural doctors by background. Also a much more politically aware group and I think that it's time we also sold the positive sides of a much shorter period of good experience.

Can I touch on professional organizations? One elephant in the room in the UK is the relationship between rural doctors and the Royal College of General Practitioners; I don't want to get involved with the rights and wrongs of this. I think it may be useful to look at lessons to be learned from other places around this, and I know that's what I spoke about at the RCGP Conference in November, by DVD presentation from Australia.[203] One of the true successes of rural medicine in Australia is that it had effective national organizations that looked after it and they were not any of the traditional ones, the rural doctors had to form their own.[204] It's now got to the point where the other organizations are bending over backwards or at least appear to be terribly supportive, and I don't think there's any doubt that in Australia both the AMA (Australian Medical Association) and the Royal Australian College of General Practitioners made serious miscalculations in not backing rural medicine as strongly as they should. I sense the same thing is happening in this country and there may be a better resolution in the light of that history. But there's no doubt that a lot of the success of Australia, the money that flows to education, that flows to practice support, to locums, came about because rural doctors did it. I think it's worth opening up the debate about the elephant in the room.

Sarah Strasser: One of the key things we identified was getting the community onside and I'll give you an example, I think, of an amazing piece of work where the doctors actually went on strike in Canada in the 1980s. This was not supported by the community and the Government stood up to the doctors

---

[203] Professor Richard Hays added: 'The RCGP National Conference in 2009 in Glasgow. There was a session held by the Rural Interest Group on whether or not to remain with the RCGP regional faculty structure where (except for Scotland and Wales) they felt rural issues did not get serious attention by the national body, or form a separate rural College, as happened in Australia. I argued for staying together.' Email to Ms Caroline Overy, 12 July 2016.

[204] The Rural Doctors Association of Australia (RDAA) and the National Rural Health Alliance were both formed in 1991, and the Australian College of Rural and Remote Medicine (ACRRM) was formed in 1997. See pages 28–9.

and it sounded like all hell broke loose.[205] We had been in Canada in the early 1980s, and when we returned in 2002, there was a huge difference in mindset; general practice had changed. With all the strikes and the change in pay systems, in general there had been huge dissatisfaction and no connection between the community and the profession, let alone between politicians, the community, and the profession. A project called Educating Future Physicians for Ontario did a fantastic, enormous consultative process with the community through focus groups, asking for submissions, trying to identify what the community wanted out of physicians.[206] There was a lot of commonality in the information that they gathered and they also asked health professional groups as well, and out of that they developed some very exciting projects that actually went on to develop some of the current leaders in medical education or health services delivery in Canada. There was a range of things, including graduate programmes and broader educational programmes, but I think that if you want to look overseas for other examples of doing things that we need to also think about the postgraduate and not just the vocational training.

Roger Strasser: Sarah just mentioned some developments in Canada because of a doctors' strike. The first Rural Doctors Associations in Australia – they still fight as to whether it was Queensland first or New South Wales first but there were doctors' strikes in both those states – and the rural doctors, of course, provide medical services in the hospitals in those states so that's how they were involved. These Rural Doctors Associations got started in about 1987. Why did they start in 1987 when the issues had been there 10, 20, 30 years before? I think the reason is the development of two pieces of communication technology: the conference call or teleconference, so that the doctors could stay in their rural communities and hold meetings in real time; and the fax machine, which meant that the doctors could develop documents and share them amongst themselves to make their case and their presentations to the political organizations. I agree with Richard Hays that it was the organizing of the rural doctors in Australia that was the beginning of making a difference for rural medicine and rural healthcare generally in Australia. To put that into

---

[205] In June 1986 the Ontario Medical Association went on strike to protest against the introduction of legislation against the billing of patients above the reimbursement level of the Ontario Hospital Insurance Plan ('extra billing'); see Meslin (1987).

[206] Professor Roger Strasser added: 'Educating Future Physicians for Ontario (EFPO) was a collaborative initiative funded by Associated Medical Services (AMS) and involving Ontario medical schools.' Note on draft transcript, 6 August 2016. See, for example, Neufeld *et al.* (1998); Maudsley *et al.* (2000).

perspective, in 1978 there had been a big national conference called 'Country Towns, Country Doctors', which was initiated by the Royal Australian College of General Practitioners.[207] The report looks lovely, but nothing happened, and nothing happened, and again nothing happened. The formation of the Rural Doctors Associations – with, I think it is fair to say, some very smart political operators leading the Associations – led to what's now referred to as the first National Rural Health Conference, which was held in 1991 in Toowoomba in Queensland.[208] I was sitting next to someone who had been at the 1978 conference. She was a Country Women's Association delegate and the issues were exactly the same and the recommendations were exactly the same, but the difference was the momentum that had been created by the Rural Doctors Associations. It led to the First Australian National Rural Health Strategy. In fact, the conference was all about debating a draft strategy that had been prepared by the organizers before the conference started. It led to the establishment of the National Rural Health Alliance, which is a national coalition of rural health-focused organizations, not just the Rural Doctors Associations from the states and the national, but other rural health interest groups. There was already a Remote Area Nurses national body that had spawned rural nurses and rural allied health organizations.[209] I think the experience of every one of those, talking about the health professional groups, was that they tried first within their parent, whether it's the College of General Practitioners or the nurses' organizations and the physiotherapy organization and so on, and they found it difficult to get the attention of the leaders in the metropolitan area. When they did, they tended to experience the response as being rather patronizing and condescending, maybe a reflection of the assumption that we know better in the city than you country bumpkins. Whatever the situation, what was certain was that the rural doctors weren't going to accept being treated that way. They made political alliances and connections and were able to make progress. In terms of the academic side of things in Australia, it was a very interesting process. Richard Hays talked about the Royal Australian College of General Practitioners and the Australian Medical Association miscalculating and making tactical errors. There was a referendum of rural GPs or rural doctors generally, I guess, in Australia in 1991/92. It was about whether the academic interests of rural doctors should be looked after under the umbrella

---

[207] Walpole (1979).

[208] See page 29 and note 26.

[209] The Council of Remote Area Nurses of Australia (CRANA).

of the Royal Australian College of General Practitioners through a faculty of rural medicine or something like that, or whether there should be a separate rural medicine college. Two-thirds of those who voted at that time voted in favour of being under the umbrella of the Royal Australian College of General Practitioners. Four years later things had gone so badly that there was the same referendum essentially, the same choice, and two-thirds voted in favour of having a separate rural college, which then happened, so the Australian College of Rural and Remote Medicine was established and has now become a major force for academic rural and remote medicine and training.[210] There's a parallel pathway for training for rural and remote practice, which has now the same status in the system in Australia as the general practice training programmes.

So that's fleshing out a bit what Richard Hays was saying happened in Australia. I can say that as I was the inaugural chair of the World Organization of National Colleges, Academies and Academic Associations of General Practitioners/Family Physicians (WONCA) Working Party on Rural Practice – WONCA's shortened name is the World Organization of Family Doctors, and members of WONCA are the College of General Practitioner equivalents in all the countries around the world. We started the Rural WONCA in 1992 – it was actually at the World WONCA Conference in Vancouver in Canada; there were a couple of sessions on rural medicine which were packed with rural doctors. The actual sessions were very badly organized and the speakers spoke for too long and the audience didn't get to say anything but they were clearly steamed up so we called an *ad hoc* meeting at lunchtime on one of the days. Seventy rural practitioners turned up so that provided the nucleus for starting the WONCA Working Party on Rural Practice.[211] To some extent this continues to this day, the debate about whether there should be a separate world organization of rural doctors or stay under the umbrella of WONCA, but I'd say that the then leadership of WONCA handled the rural doctors in a different way, so we were able to stay under the umbrella of WONCA. Over the years I have visited many countries, including this one, and been invited to speak at meetings about these issues. I've just come from Norway, but before that, in December 2009, I was invited to Brazil, because the equivalent of the College of General Practitioners in Brazil, the president, has realized that they've had general practice or family medicine recognized as a specialty for 20 years but there's no recognition of rural medicine. I was invited to speak

---

[210] See www.acrrm.org.au (accessed 23 August 2016).

[211] See note 8.

at their National Conference of General Practitioners to present the case for rural medicine being recognized as a specialty. This was a more positive experience than many because it was actually the leadership of the organization who invited me to speak and invited local rural doctors to talk about their experiences to start that process. Many other times it's been set up actually as a debate or as a confrontation and then there's been local resolution in that country. It sounds like in this country the debate continues or at least the resolution from the past with the Rural Standing Committee isn't meeting the needs of the rural practitioners now and there's a new sense that this has to be addressed in the UK.

Baird: Well, thinking about the UK, Jim Cox, from your perspective the College [Royal College of General Practitioners] works for you but you actually are quite close to your faculty and you've got a faculty that's responsive to your needs. The engagement of rural general practice with government and with our own organizational bodies, which includes the BMA and the RCGP, is very poor and I'll give an example of each aspect. Firstly Iain McNicol and I tried to engage with the Remote and Rural Health Education Alliance, which was a Scottish organization, with a statutory requirement to do so and I think it took us four months to organize a meeting and we organized three outcomes and so far, I think that as far as we're concerned, Iain's made progress.[212] In terms of the College, the fact is that the faculty structure of which the College is signed up to does not represent rural general practitioners in any way, shape, or form. Attempts to get the College to resolve that problem by producing a non-geographical faculty have failed, and their refusal to accept the lack of faculty representation is an absolute disgrace and a shame on the Royal College of General Practitioners over the last 20 or so years. I'm not sure what the way out is, but certainly I don't think we should exclude the Australian solution of having to go it alone. That would not be, given the last 17 years of effort trying to engage with the College, my primary wish but I suspect that's one thing to do. The BMA no longer looks at rural issues, although there used to be a rural subcommittee. So I think representation at all of these levels is a major and almost totally un-addressed issue, except possibly to give credit where credit's

---

[212] 'The Remote and Rural Healthcare Educational Alliance is part of NHS Education for Scotland (NES) … [working] across all the remote, rural and island areas of Scotland helping to coordinate remote and rural healthcare education development and support education and training for the remote, rural and island workforce … [Its] aims are to increase access to affordable, sustainable education, training and development opportunities'; www.rrheal.scot.nhs.uk/what-we-do.aspx (accessed 28 June 2016).

due to the College, at least it paid some lip service to it, but my feeling and the feeling of most of my colleagues is that that is where the big gap has lain in the past and will lie in the future.

Douglas: Could I make a very brief comment? I'll try to be brief. On balance, I think the Royal College of General Practitioners has done more good than harm for general practice in the UK since it was formed in the 1950s and for remote and rural general practitioners as part of that. The problem isn't going to go away – we've talked a lot about the 2004 contract and the change to postgraduate and medical training across the whole of the UK recently with the Postgraduate Medical Educational Training Board. Now everybody who wants to become a general practitioner in the UK must be a member of the College.[213] The great divide-and-rule thing that occurred for my generation – half the lobby were in the BMA and the other half were in the Royal College of General Practitioners – is now not going to be. The other thing that has happened is that the training programme is now called the general practice specialty training, so the UK, top-of-the-tree board, the General Medical Council, is now talking about general practice as a specialty. In other words generalism as a specialty. I think we can learn from the Australian experience; the Australians have got quite a lot out of splitting the two things and going away with a separate remote and rural faculty, but I think there have been disadvantages and it would be a big problem if we allowed a divide-and-rule situation here and I think we're better at sticking with trying to work within the college model. Whether things are called faculties or whether they are called working groups or forums or whatever in colleges – this maybe is a technical thing for non-UK people – but Royal Colleges have antibodies to the word 'faculty' because faculties mean if you have a faculty of paediatrics it becomes a Royal College of Paediatrics, if you have a faculty of anaesthetists it becomes a Royal College of Anaesthetists, so the 'F' word in a Royal College causes big problems for them. I think you've got to be more politically astute in this country and not use the 'F' word, I think we've got to use maybe the word 'forum' or something.

We talk about education and I want to talk about the important thing in remote and rural healthcare of sustainability of CPD (continuing professional development) in remote practitioners and want to celebrate in particular the BASICS movement (the British Association of Immediate Care Systems), which started in England in 1977 and has been done particularly well in Scotland

---

[213] In 2007 a new mandatory MRCGP assessment was introduced for all doctors wanting to become GPs.

under somebody who unfortunately we should have probably tried to get invited to the meeting but isn't here, Colville Laird.[214] That has set up a model of immediate care education, in other words GPs living in rural communities going to road accidents, going to people with heart attacks, going to children with breathing difficulties or whatever and feeling confident about that. The model of that educational system has been to take the educational package out to the rural community, in other words setting up in the local village hall, the local hotel, and it's all about trying to allow people to feel confident in things that they don't see very often, so it's all about skill acquisition and maintenance of skills so that people can be confident. One of the reasons that people leave rural communities is because if they don't see something regularly they become worried about it; this whole method of training, where you take the training into the community, giving the people a recharge of their practical skills, is a positive method of keeping people in post.

I also want to briefly mention the business about certification: the balance between certification and training. Training is a good thing. Certification has got good points and bad points about it. We've got to make sure that we don't have so much certification that we create barriers for going into rural practice and we've got to be careful about pedantic models: 'Unless you've done so many of these you can't do it anymore.' I think we need modern models of adult professional peer appraisal and self-diagnosis by the professional, by the doctor in what their skills are and what their educational needs are because we can start tying people into boxes and big centralist things. The last sentence is a plea for rural training within rural communities and, yes, certification and qualifications are a good idea, but we have to be careful that we don't go too far with that and produce barriers.

Parry: The Association of Rural Surgeons of India was formed because a group of Indian surgeons were so concerned at the divide between urban surgery and rural surgery that they formed their own association and my colleague, Jill Donnelly from Hereford, attends their annual meeting and comes back deeply enthused.[215]

---

[214] For BASICS, see note 136. Dr Colville Laird is a GP in Auchterarder, and Medical Director of BASICS Scotland. He has run immediate care courses in Scotland since 1993.

[215] The Association of Rural Surgeons of India (ARSI) was launched in 1993 and 'aims to take appropriate surgery to the doorsteps of the rural population' (www.arsi-india.org/arsi_origin.htm, accessed 29 June 2016). Jill Donnelly is a consultant breast surgeon at the County Hospital, Wye Valley NHS Trust, Hereford.

Pereira Gray: Thank you very much, that's a very positive note to finish with. We have got the last item on the agenda – which is the very important bit – we must make a place for about taking it forward. We've had a very good couple of sessions but the real question again is, how do we take this forward and how would you feel as a group that it's best recorded or studied and what future do you have in mind?

Douglas: The first thing I would like to say is 'thank you' to this group for inviting the next generation. I think that's innovative to get David Hogg here as part of the next generation and I think we've got to move with what the requirements of the next generation are in trying to capture and record history and professional identity and so on. We've got to use social networking websites and all that modern technology, for trying to capture a lot of this.

Cox: Could we hear from Tilli? Having listened to this and being the most experienced person in this process, could you guide us? What are the options?

Tansey: I must say I'm very relieved that something that Roger Strasser said earlier today is clearly wrong, because he did say that all rural GPs are very self-effacing. It's been fascinating listening although I'm not very sure how much history there's been here. There's been an awful lot of contemporary issues with historical roots and I think those historical roots are worth investigating. I jotted down some notes, some words like 'professional identity', 'sustainability and training issues', 'service provision', and 'status'. These rang a bell with me so at the tea break I looked at my notes and exactly the same four criteria came up at a previous Witness Seminar, one which we ran on clinical pharmacology, and those were all complaints that clinical pharmacologists were making.[216] I do agree and I think this issue of the biomedical orientated university, this almost molecular way of looking at medical education in this country is astonishing. I would love to know more about Keele and what the drivers were, particularly for the rural medicine project; so that is one specific question. It's also important to hear the non-medical, the other voices, Roger Strasser mentioned the nurses in one sentence, we haven't really heard anything about the nurses, and certainly not from the nurses. We've not heard much about the patients, although we've heard of them in car parks and getting on helicopters. There's an awful lot here, we've not heard anything at all about technology, apart from the helicopter and the fax machine.[217] There's a lot of history that could be usefully examined,

---

[216] Reynolds and Tansey (eds) (2008).

[217] See the discussion on technology on pages 52–4 and 63–6.

that might actually be useful for the future generations of practitioners, and for you as well to actually consolidate your own experience.[218] The international globalization aspect of this particularly interests me, I think that is something very powerful. Is there something we could capture there? Is this something we could try to work up a proposal to getting funding for? Is it something that people are interested in or some of you are interested in? So what kind of histories? How do we get it? Who does it and what is its purpose?

Hogg: Can I come in on the technology side of things? This is an idea in which I'm particularly interested, particularly in terms of networking, both for trainees and rural GPs; I'll keep it concise because I'm aware of time. Skype, a group of GP Registrars that I set up, have had a very successful session, in fact we've had two sessions now. We linked up a trainee in Lochgilphead, a trainee in Derbyshire, a trainee in Sheffield, a trainee in Oxfordshire, and myself, in Glasgow.[219] The cost? Free. I think that needs to be highlighted. We're actually doing a lot of work in terms of practice-based small-group learning and trying to pioneer some of that, although again there is some work to be done. If we're looking for good qualitative, anecdotal contributions from across rural areas, I think we need to embrace technology in that way because it is becoming increasingly easy to use. Although I appreciate coming into London, it has been relatively easy for me, for the real guys on the ground who are often stuck in those areas it offers a fantastic opportunity for them to contribute.

Sarah Strasser: I wondered if there was going to be an opportunity for this project to spread a little because I would put in a plea for you to get some stories from the families of rural GPs because it was quite a different way of life. As a child growing up with both my parents who were rural GPs and their practice was in our house and it was very much a fishbowl experience, not that we were familiar with that term at the time, but it's very interesting and I know that some of the rural GP family stories from Australia have been fascinating and it might complement what you've got here.

---

[218] Professor Sir Denis Pereira Gray wrote: 'The RCGP Heritage Committee, Chairman Dr Bill Reith FRCPEd FRCGP, meets regularly to consider the archives and heritage items of the College and to promote its history. The RCGP Archivist, Dr Sharon Messenger, attends the Committee, organises heritage events, like the RCGP plaques of leading GPs, and runs exhibitions and open days.' Letter to Ms Caroline Overy, 19 August 2016.

[219] Dr Hogg wrote: 'Skype worked with audio only when having more than 2 people. However this still worked fairly well, providing it was chaired assertively in an organised manner.' Email to Mrs Lois Reynolds, 5 July 2010.

Baird: I connect very strongly with the idea that it should be families. A few years ago there was a keynote speech at the Royal College of General Practitioners' AGM by a US family doctor who told a story of his father. One of the things that resonated with me was leaving his mother with a smashed Bakelite handset to answer the telephone with because he'd smashed it down in rage before going out to see the patient; that I do remember happened to my mother. Home and surgery were profoundly connected and I'm sure Jim Cox and Iain McNicol remember well. My uncle, Hugh Baird (subsequently a founding member of BASICS and Scottish BASICS' first chair), took over from my grandfather. He upset many patients, because he got rid of the lady who answered the door to let the patients in. The reality of that was that the patients had to come through past the living area and too many items of furniture and ornamentation had gone astray so the door was locked and somebody had to show you into the waiting room so that nothing got lifted, but it was regarded as a retrograde step when Agnes disappeared from the surgery. I do remember the first time I ever saw my mother and father arguing, because for the first time in two years there were four kids in the car who were ready to go on holiday and the front door had been left unlocked for some years and wasn't able to be locked before we went on holiday. I remember too the respect tradesmen had for the commitment that the GP made to the community and came out on a Sunday and fixed the door lock so we could all disappear happily on holiday. This connection with your personal family and other people's family was quite appropriate. I think it's perhaps worth recording historically, apart from the organizational stuff, about how actually it was because I think there was no work–life balance; it was the same thing. I think that has pretty well completely disappeared. Our surgery moved from the house two or three years ago and I don't miss the doorbell going at all.

Roger Strasser: I'd like to thank Tilli for bringing us together; this has been a wonderful discussion. I believe very much that this is the very beginning of developing a history of rural medicine and rural medical education. Quite a number of themes have come through, which bear exploring in more depth, and some others haven't been much more than just raised – technology is one, women in rural practice is another, there are quite a few others – so I hope that this is the beginning of a process of working in different ways and together in some ways, and maybe in other directions to ensure that a history of rural medicine is developed. In five years' time, when you go to the Wellcome Library catalogue, you will see many publications that provide a documentation, not only of what happened, but also a sense, as our discussions have been, very much of interpretations. I think Tilli mentioned the contemporary issues and their historical roots; it seems to me that one of the important values of history is the understanding of how the current situation has come about, because if we want to change the current situation we don't want to make the same mistakes as the past or to fall in to traps that we would know about if we understood the history. I'd like to see this as a dynamic developmental process that will facilitate the future development of rural medicine and rural medical education.

Tansey: May I suggest that in the first instance you all think about how you'd like future plans developed. What I would not want to encourage is to start something that is going to fade away and that will be it; it would have to be sustainable.

Pereira Gray: That seems to strike a very intensive note, Tilli, looking round the room. Well, I think time is coming to an end. I would like to say, as the listener here, that it's been very stimulating for me and I think it's been a very vigorous discussion and I agree with Tilli that it has touched on what she called 'contemporary issues', the historical analysis, but we did get some of that too, particularly earlier on in the first session. We are very grateful to the Wellcome Trust History of Twentieth Century Medicine Group, who facilitated the whole thing; it was a vision of yours and I think, Tilli, we ought to thank you and your team. I'm very encouraged if you think there's a way that can take this forward in the future.

Tansey: And, of course, thank you very much, Denis, for chairing this meeting and keeping everyone under control.

Biographical notes[*]

Professor Ivar Aaraas

PhD (b. 1944) grew up on a farm in the countryside in the south of Norway. After medical graduation in Oslo in 1969 he headed towards Northern Norway for internship. Since then he has been living and working in the northern part of the country most of the time. After five years in different hospital specialties he turned to work as a GP and rural medical doctor for 15 years. Since 1987, his main affiliation has been with University of Tromsø, the Arctic University of Norway, partially combined with clinical and public health work. In 1998 he defended a PhD about use and usefulness of general practitioners' hospitals (cottage hospitals) in a northern rural county. From 2006 until retirement in 2014 he was professor and head of the Norwegian National Centre of Rural Medicine in Tromsø. A main focus of Aaraas' teaching and research has been the importance of communication and coordination both between patient and doctor and between the different levels of healthcare. A particular topic, with several written and oral educational contributions, has been how to cope with medical uncertainty, including prevention and handling of medical errors

Dr A Gordon Baird

MBChB MRCOG FRCGP (b. 1952) graduated in Glasgow in 1976. The third generation of West Galloway rural GPs, he succeeded his father as a GP principal, serving BASICS, the RNLI, an MOD range, and a community hospital. In addition to GP duties and being a rural hospital practitioner, he was clinical lead for a GP hospital with 16,000 A&E attendances annually and 1,200 acute medical admissions. This hospital was the first community hospital in the UK to deliver thrombolysis for myocardial infarction and for stroke. A founding member of the Rural Practice task force of the RCGP and chairman for four years between 2005 and 2008, he contributed to *Rural Healthcare* (Cox and Mungall (eds) (1998)), and 'Rural deprivation' in *Working with Vulnerable Groups: A clinical handbook for GPs*. (Gill, Wright, and Brew (eds) (2014). He discovered a new presentation of

[*] Contributors are asked to supply details; other entries are compiled from conventional biographical sources.

Lyme disease as proof of endemic disease besides publishing on deprivation and access issues.

Professor Petar Bulat

MD MSc PhD (b. 1961) graduated in medicine from the University of Belgrade in 1986, and obtained his MSc in toxicology in 1991, and PhD in toxicology in 1994. He has been employed by the University of Belgrade Faculty of Medicine and the Serbian Institute of Occupational Health since 1989. He is responsible for occupational health teaching as well as for running a clinical department on occupational toxicology, and since 2012 has held the position of Vice-Dean responsible for clinical teaching at the University of Belgrade Faculty of Medicine. He was Assistant Director of the Serbian Institute of Occupational Health (2001–2009) and was Republic of Serbia Assistant Minister of Health responsible for foreign affairs (2011–2012). From 2006 to 2012 he was Secretary of ICOH Scientific Committee on Rural Health, from 2006 to 2015 he was Vice-President of the European Association of Schools of Occupational Medicine, and from 2009 onward he has been Vice-President of the Serbian Society of Toxicology.

Professor (Alan) Bruce Chater

MB BS Hons FACRRM DRANZCOG (Advanced) FRACGP (b. 1956) is from Queensland, Australia, where he is Medical Superintendent with Right to Private Practice in Theodore, Chair of the Statewide Rural and Remote Clinical Network, Head of the Discipline of Rural and Remote Medicine at University of Queensland, Secretary of the international WONCA (World Organization of Family Doctors) Working Party on Rural Practice and on the Australian Independent Hospital Pricing Authority Board. He was the founding convenor of the Rural Doctors Associations of Queensland and Australia and the founding Chair of the Australian National Rural Health Alliance. Performing these roles from his rural base of Theodore, Dr Chater remains grounded in the needs of rural communities. His practice since 1981 as the Medical Superintendent with Right to Private Practice in the small town of Theodore is an exemplar of rural practice, encompassing services including surgery and obstetrics, general practice and inpatient care, ultrasonography and X-rays, private practice, and hospital practice.

Professor Ian Couper

BA MBBCh MFamMed FCFP(SA)
(b. 1961) qualified in medicine at
the University of the Witwatersrand
(Wits) and held hospital posts
in Port Elizabeth and Manguzi
Hospital. From 2000 to 2002
he was Senior Lecturer in the
Department of Family Medicine,
MEDUNSA (Medical University
of Southern Africa), and Senior
Specialist (Family Physician) in the
Odi District, North West Province.
In 2002 he was appointed Professor
of Rural Health at the University of
the Witwatersrand, Johannesburg,
where he was director of the Wits
Centre for Rural Health, and
Head of the Clinical Unit (family
medicine) in the North West
Provincial Department of Health.
He held this post until 2016, when
he was appointed Professor of
Rural Health and Director of the
Ukwanda Centre for Rural Health,
Faculty of Medicine and Health
Sciences, at Stellenbosch University.
He was active in the formation
of the Rural Doctors Association
of Southern Africa (RuDASA) in
1997, and chaired the international
Working Party on Rural Practice of
the World Organization of Family
Doctors from 2007 to 2013. He
was a member of the national
task team to develop the clinical
associate programme in South
Africa, and led the development of

such training at Wits. He has been
involved in supporting medical
education initiatives in a number
of African countries.

Dr Jim Cox

OBE DL MD FRCP(Edin)
FRCGP (b. 1950) was a rural
general practitioner in Caldbeck,
Cumbria, Medical Director of
Cumbria Ambulance Service, and
founder chairman of the Royal
College of General Practitioners
Rural Practice Group. He co-
edited *Rural Healthcare* (Cox and
Mungall (eds) (1998)) and was a
board member of the Countryside
Agency and Commission for Rural
Communities.

Dr James Douglas

MBChB MD FRCGP FRCPE
DOccMed (b. 1951) graduated in
medicine from the University of
Aberdeen in 1975. He completed
his vocational training for UK
General Practice in 1980 and
became a partner in Tweeddale
Medical Practice, Fort William, in
the Scottish rural Highlands where
he remains as a clinical scientist
within his rural community. He has
wide-ranging clinical and research
interests, which began with diving
medicine, and publications on
emergency treatment methods and
diving long-term health hazards.
He was the first doctor to describe
occupational health in salmon

farming and published the first research on salmon processing as a new cause of occupational asthma, which became the subject for his MD thesis as a clinical GP. He then researched flu diagnosis and flu immunization in clinical practice. His current rural research interest is Lyme borelliosis in his community. He has been involved in professional standards and leadership within the Royal College of General Practitioners and NHS Education Scotland. He has an interest in international rural health and education as a member of WONCA and has contributed to the medical education literature. He chaired the Dewar Centenary medical history group in 2012.

Emeritus Professor John Davis Hamilton

AM OBE MBBS FRCP(Can) FRCP(Lon) (b. 1937) studied medicine at the Middlesex Hospital, receiving his medical degree in 1960. From 1962 to 1964 he was Medical Officer at St Francis Hospital, Zambia, and from 1965 to 1969 he carried out research in gastroenterology at St Bartholomew's Hospital, London. In 1969 he was appointed Director of Gastroenterology and Chair of Curriculum and Student Selection in the Faculty of Health Sciences at McMaster University, Canada, where he

remained until 1978, when he moved to the Faculty of Health Sciences at the University of Ilorin, Nigeria, as Chair of Curriculum Committee. Between 1981 and 1983 he worked in the Population, Health and Nutrition Division, World Bank in Washington DC, after which he moved to Australia and in 1984 was appointed Dean of the Faculty of Medicine and Health Science, Newcastle University, Australia. There he was on the Hunter Area Health Board and Chair of the Appointment and Credentials Committee; Foundation Chair of the Australian Medical Council Accreditation Committee; Chair of the Australian Quality of Health Care Study; Chair of the Committee on Women in Medicine; and Chair of Rural Undergraduate Steering Committee (RUSC); WHO Consultant in Medical Education; Chair of the Diarrheal Diseases Control Program; and on the Board of the WHO's SEARO TROPMED Program. From 2000 to 2005 he was Academic Director of the medical school of Durham University, after which he became Professor Emeritus at the University of Newcastle, and Chair of the clinical years four and five. He assists in medical schools, most recently in Nigeria, South Africa, and Iran. In 2006 he received an OBE for services to international medical education, and in 2012 became a Member of the Order of Australia (AM) for services to medicine and tertiary education and indigenous health. He has honorary doctorates from Newcastle (Australia), Newcastle (UK), and Walter Sisulu University (South Africa).

Professor Richard Hays
MBBS PhD MD FRACGP FACRRM FRCGP FAMEE FAcadMedEd FHEA (b. 1953) was a rural procedural general practitioner in northern Australia before becoming a teacher and education researcher, with a career focus on developing new or change-managing established programmes and institutional structures in regional and rural communities. He gained higher qualifications in educational psychology and medical education, and has been the Head or Dean of four medical schools in Australia and the United Kingdom: Foundation Dean, James Cook University, Australia (1999–2005); Head, Keele Medical School, United Kingdom (2006–2010); Dean, Faculty of Health, Bond University, Australia (2010–2014); Dean of Medicine, University of Tasmania (2015–2016). He has been a consultant to other developments in Europe, South East Asia, the Western Pacific region, and Canada. He has contributed to international medical education quality assurance and accreditation processes, through the Australian Medical Council, the General Medical Council, and the World Federation of Medical Education. Along the way he has been awarded about three million Australian dollars in competitive research and development grants and has published about 100 research papers, 150 other journal articles, 16 book chapters and 9 books, primarily on assessment, curriculum design, and educational quality assurance, all with a strong rural flavour.

Dr David Hogg
BSc (MedSci) MBChB DCH (b. 1981) qualified in medicine from Glasgow in 2005. Foundation training in Stirling and Glasgow led him to GP training in Ayrshire, where he was a GP registrar. He became a GP Rural Fellow on the Isle of Arran in August 2010 and one of the GP principals in April 2013. He set up the website RuralGP.com in 2008 and has maintained it since. He is a member of Arran Mountain Rescue Team and Honorary Senior Clinical Lecturer in Remote & Rural Medicine at Glasgow University.

Professor Geoffrey Hudson

DPhil (b. 1962) studied history at McMaster University (BA Hons, MA) and received his doctorate from Oxford University in 1996. After a Research Fellowship at the Wellcome Trust Centre for the History of Medicine at University College London (1997–1999), he became Programs Director at the Hannah Institute for the History of Medicine (Associated Medical Services, Toronto, Ontario) in 1999. In the 2003–2004 academic year he was Acting Director, History of Medicine Unit, Faculty of Health Sciences, McMaster University, Hamilton, ON, and in 2004 was appointed Assistant Professor at the Northern Ontario School of Medicine (Faculty of Medicine, Lakehead and Laurentian Universities). Since 2008, he has been Associate Professor in the History of Medicine, Human Sciences Division in the Medical School, as well as Adjunct Professor in Lakehead's History Department. His research focuses on the social history of medicine, war and medicine, as well as the history of disability. Hudson's teaching activities since joining the Medical School includes service as a coordinator for the module (unique in the world) in which all students are placed in indigenous communities across Northern Ontario.

Professor Victor Inem

MBBS (b. 1955) is a professor of family medicine and primary healthcare. He received his MBBS degree in 1980 from the University of Lagos, Nigeria. He became a fellow of the National Postgraduate Medical College of Nigeria in 1989 and of the West African College of Physicians in 1992. He specializes in rural remote and riverine medicine and his involvement in participatory research has got him closer to the grassroots. His other research interests include the reproductive health of families and child health. He has lectured in these areas at Delta and Ebonyi state universities from 2004 to 2013, and has worked as a consultant, principal investigator, and facilitator for local and international health organizations, including the Federal Ministry of Health, NPHCDA, WHO, UNICEF, and USAID. He was a member of the Nigerian Government vision 20/20 Health thematic group in 2009. He is a member of several professional bodies and was formerly the Secretary General of the Nigerian Medical Association (1996–1998) and the Association of General and

Private Medical Practitioners of Nigeria (1987–1995). He has been a member of the WONCA Rural Working Party since 1992. He has published over 70 papers in peer-reviewed journals, is the author of the book *Foundational Knowledge for the Practice of Family Medicine in West Africa*, and is editor of several national and international academic and professional journals. He is at present a lecturer at his alma mater in the department of Community Health and Primary Care, College of Medicine, University of Lagos; a pioneer coach and mentor to the prestigious Nigeria diploma in family medicine programme; and also an honorary consultant to the Lagos University Teaching Hospital and former acting director of Primary Health Care Centre, Pakoto.

Dr Oleg Kravtchenko

MD (b. 1963) is the son of a Russian army officer. He graduated from Moscow Medical Academy in 1986, and specialized in ENT surgery at Central Postgraduate University, Moscow, and Eppendorf University, Hamburg. He practised at the Central Clinical Hospital in Moscow until 1998 when he moved to Norway. He studied at Oslo University and then practised at the Nordland Central Hospital, ENT department, and later the Obstetrics and Gynaecology

department. He specialized as a GP in 2002 and worked in rural practice in Meløy community, Nordland, until summer 2012, when he became co-owner at the Fredensborg Klinikken, Nordland. He works as a full-time GP and is an Overseas Fellow of the Royal Society of Medicine, London, and Vice-President of EURIPA, WONCA.

Dr Iain McNicol

MBE MBChB CCFP(Can) (b. 1949), a third generation doctor in the family. He graduated MBChB in Glasgow in 1974 and CCFP(Can) in Memorial University of Newfoundland in 1978. He worked in a cancer clinic in Germany in 1971 and a remote psychiatric hospital in Northern Ontario in 1972. After house jobs in Inverness and Glasgow, he was a trainee in Woodside HC and Bearsden, Family Medicine Residency in Newfoundland with Keith Hodgkin, John Ross, Paul Patey, and John Lewis. He was a GP on Flotta, Orkney from 1979 to 1981, then a single-handed practitioner in Appin and Lismore from 1981 to 2009. McNicol was Medical Adviser to Glensanda Super Quarry from 1985 to 2011, and carried out locums throughout Argyll and the Isles in retirement from 2009 to 2014. He was Scottish BASICS Board member

(1986–2006) and Chair (1992–1994); Chair of Argyll Immediate Care Scheme (1992–2009); Chair of the Inducement Practitioners' Association (Latterly Remote P A) (1989–2003), thereafter Life President; and Member of the Primary Care Solutions Group (RARARI) (2001–2003). He was awarded the MBE in 2005. He is married with four children, and his hobbies include history, sailing, walking, community enterprise (Chair of Appin Community Cooperative 1983–2016), and writing.

Professor Sir Eldryd Parry
KCMG OBE FRCP (b. 1930) has been visiting professor at the London School of Hygiene and Tropical Medicine since 1985 and from 1989 to 2007 was chairman of the Tropical Health and Education Trust, which works with medical schools and other training institutions in Africa to provide services relevant to local needs. He worked at University College Hospital, Ibadan, Nigeria from 1960 to 1963 and at Haile Selassie I University, Addis Ababa, Ethiopia, from 1966 to 1969; he was Professor of Medicine at Ahmadu Bello University, Zaria, Nigeria, from 1969 to 1977; Foundation Dean of the Faculty of Health Sciences at the University of Ilorin, Nigeria, from 1977 to 1980, and Dean and Professor of Medicine at the School of Medical Sciences, Kumasi, from 1980 to 1985. In 1985 he became director of the Wellcome Tropical Institute (formerly the Wellcome Museum of Medical Science) until 1990. See Parry and Ikeme (1966); Parry (ed.) (1976).

Dr Tanja Pekez-Pavlisko
MD (b. 1961) finished medical school at the University of Banja Luka in 1985 and moved to Zagreb in 1989. She was a resident in emergency medicine (but didn't finish because of the war) and carried out a postgraduate course in clinical pharmacology, a postgraduate course in emergency medicine and family medicine, and a PhD course at the medical school at Zagreb University. Before the residency in family medicine, she had great experience in pre-hospital emergency care. She was an ALS (advanced life support) instructor and was ITLS (International Trauma Life Support) Medical Director for Croatia, participating in mass casualties courses. She was President of the organizing committee of the KoHOM (Croatian Family Physicians Coordination) congresses in 2013 and 2014; President of organizing committee of WONCA Rural Health Congress in Dubrovnik in 2015; President of EURIPA;

and Vice-Chair of the WONCA Working Party on Rural Practice. She is also a reviewer on World and European family medicine conferences. Her special interests include rural medicine, domestic violence, patient safety, education, emergency medicine, and palliative care.

Professor Sir Denis Pereira Gray

OBE HonDSc HonDM FRCP FRCGP FMedSci (b. 1935) was a general practitioner in the St Leonard's Practice Exeter for 38 years (1962–2000), following his father and grandfather. He established the first postgraduate university department of general practice in Europe at Exeter University. He was elected Chairman of Council of the RCGP, Chairman of the Joint Committee of Postgraduate Training for General Practice and later President of the College. He is the only British GP to have been elected Chairman of the Trustees of the Nuffield Trust and the Academy of Medical Royal Colleges. His writings include four books and over 200 articles. He has been awarded three gold medals from professional bodies and three Honorary Doctorates from British universities.

Professor Maja Račić

MD MsD PhD (b. 1972) qualified in medicine in Kragujevac, Serbia, in 1997. After a residency in family medicine in Banja Luka, Bosnia, from 1999 to 2002, she obtained a Master's degree in Belgrade, Serbia, in 2005 and received her PhD from the Medical Faculty, East Sarajevo, Bosnia, in 2007. From 1997 to 2004 she worked in a family medicine practice at the Health Centre, Sokolac, working as a medical assistant for Médicins sans Frontières in 1999, and between 2004 and 2006 she was Manager of the Health Centre Stari Grad, East Sarajevo. From 2005 to 2008 she was a Lecturer in the Family Medicine Department at the University of East Sarajevo, and from 2008 to 2012 she was Head of that department. She is currently Vice-Dean for science and research, Faculty of Medicine, University of East Sarajevo and in family practice in Kosevsko Brdo, Sarajevo.

Ms Jane Randall-Smith

MA MSc (b. 1953) read Natural Sciences at Girton College, University of Cambridge, and gained an MSc in Food Science at the University of Leeds. She went on to work as a food scientist for a major food retailer, in central Government, and in the European Commission as a scientific expert. Following relocation to mid-Wales, she became technical director of a legal and technical consultancy to the food industry. After a career break, she had a complete change of direction and was involved in the establishment and subsequent management of the Institute of Rural Health, an academic centre of excellence in rural health and well-being. In 2013, she was appointed the first Chief Officer of the newly established Healthwatch Shropshire, a local consumer champion for health and social care in Shropshire and part of an England-wide network.

Professor James Rourke

MD CCFP(EM) MCISci FCFP FRRMS FCAHS LLD (b. 1952) grew up on a farm and attended a one-room, rural public school. He was an active rural family physician (including obstetrics and emergency work) in Goderich, Ontario for 25 years with his wife and partner Dr Leslie Rourke. He became Professor of Family Medicine and Assistant Dean of Rural and Regional Medicine at the University of Western Ontario and founded SWORM (the Southwestern Ontario Rural Medicine Education Research and Development Unit), which has now evolved to the Distributed Education Network of the Schulich School of Medicine and Dentistry, Western University. He served as

Dean of Medicine and Professor of Family Medicine at Memorial University of Newfoundland from 2004 to 2016. Since moving to Newfoundland and Labrador, Professor Rourke has travelled extensively to visit the medical school's teaching sites. This has included visits to conduct medical clinics in rural communities in Newfoundland and Labrador. He was Chair (2009–2011) of the Association of Faculties of Medicine of Canada (AFMC) and a leader in the Future of Medical Education in Canada projects. He was Chair (2011–2016) of the Canadian Medical Forum (CMF), and is Chair (2012–present) of the AMEE Aspire-to-Excellence Panel on Social Accountability of Medical Schools. He was Chair (2004–2007) of the WONCA Working Party in Rural Practice. As Project Director, Medical Education Design Team (2000–2001) for the Northern Ontario (Rural) Medical School Project proposal, Professor Rourke was very involved in the initial development work that led to approval to build the Northern Ontario School of Medicine. He has had over 100 medical journal articles published. He has received many honours and awards, including the University of Western Ontario: Honorary Degree Doctor of Laws, honoris causa (LLD);

Society of Rural Physicians of Canada: Rural Leadership Award; College of Family Physicians of Canada: D I Rice Merit Award and W Victor Johnston Award; College of Physicians and Surgeons of Ontario Council Award 'to honour outstanding Ontario physicians who have demonstrated excellence and come closest to meeting society's vision of an "ideal physician"'.

Dr Joseph (Jo) Scott-Jones

MMSc (General Practice) DipClinEd DipSportsMed DipObs DipGeriatricMed FDivRHM FRNZCGP MRCGP (b. 1963) graduated MBChB from the University of Sheffield in 1986, and completed his GP training in Bristol in 1990. He settled in Opotiki in New Zealand in 1991 as a rural GP. He was past Chair of the New Zealand Rural General Practice Network; appointed Senior Lecturer in the Auckland University Department of General Practice; inaugural Chair of the Rural Health Alliance Aotearoa New Zealand 2012; and Chair of the Rural Faculty of the Royal New Zealand College of General Practice.

Professor Roger Strasser

AM MBBS BMedSc MClSc DipRANZCOG DA(Eng) FRACGP FACRRM FRCGP(Hon) (b. 1952) graduated in medicine from Monash University (Australia) in 1977, undertook general practice training in Australia and Britain, and obtained his MClSc in Family Medicine from the University of Western Ontario (Canada) in 1985. Following his return to Australia, he entered rural general practice in Moe, Victoria and in 1986 became Gippsland Regional Coordinator for GP training and joined Monash University as senior lecturer. He led development of the Monash Master of Family Medicine program. In 1992, Professor Strasser was appointed Australia's first Professor of Rural Health and Head of the Centre for Rural Health, which evolved in 2001 to become the Monash University School of Rural Health. He moved to Canada in 2002 to be founding Dean of the Northern Ontario School of Medicine. Between 1992 and 2004, he had an international role as inaugural Chair of the Working Party on Rural Practice of WONCA. Recognition of his contributions includes: Fellow of WONCA (2004); Fellow of Monash University (2011); and Special Prince Mahidol Award for Outstanding Health Professional Educators recognizing visionary leadership that has changed paradigms of learning (2014).

Professor Sarah Strasser

MBBS FRACGP FACRRM
(b. 1955) graduated from the
Royal Free Hospital, University of
London in 1981. She trained as a
GP in Cornwall and the Isles of
Scilly and completed her training
at the University of Western
Ontario, Canada. She subsequently
worked in rural general practice
in Australia and Canada with an
increasing senior leadership and
academic role. Professor Strasser
established a number of new
education programmes in both
undergraduate and postgraduate
medical education in Australia and
Canada, with a particular focus
on community engagement and
social accountability. Notably she
helped establish the foundation for
the Flinders University Northern
Territory Medical Program
(NTMP); and from 2010 to
2013 she was appointed as the
inaugural Associate Dean and
Head of Faculty for Flinders NT.
She returned to Canada in 2014 to
take on a new role as the Associate
Vice-President Academics and
Interprofessional Practice at Health
Sciences North, the Academic
Teaching Centre for the Northern
Ontario School of Medicine in
North Eastern Ontario, and in
August 2016 was appointed head
of the University of Queensland
School of Rural Health based in
Toowoomba. Her research interests
include rural and remote health
workforce, gender and equity
issues, and social accountability.
She is married to Roger Strasser and
they have five children, of whom
two have taken up medicine.

Professor Tilli Tansey

OBE PhD PhD DSc HonMD
HonFRCP FMedSci (b. 1953)
graduated in zoology from the
University of Sheffield in 1974,
and obtained her PhD in *Octopus*
neuropharmacology in 1978. She
worked as a neuroscientist in the
Stazione Zoologica Naples, the
Marine Laboratory in Plymouth,
the MRC Brain Metabolism Unit,
Edinburgh, and was a Multiple
Sclerosis Society Research Fellow
at St Thomas' Hospital, London
(1983–1986). After a short
sabbatical break at the Wellcome
Institute for the History of
Medicine (WIHM), she took a
second PhD in medical history
on the career of Sir Henry Dale,
and became a member of the
academic staff of the WIHM, later
the Wellcome Trust Centre for the
History of Medicine at UCL. She
became Professor of the History
of Modern Medical Sciences
at UCL in 2007 and moved to
Queen Mary, University of London
(QMUL), with the same title, in
2010. With the late Sir Christopher
Booth she created the History

of Twentieth Century Medicine Group in the early 1990s, now the History of Modern Biomedicine Research Group at QMUL.

Dr John Wynn-Jones

BSc MBBS FRCGP DRCOG DCH (b. 1951) has been a rural GP in Wales for over 30 years. He has now retired from his full-time practice but still continues to work part time. He trained at Guy's Hospital London (1969–1975) but after finishing his GP training returned to his native Wales to work in a rural practice in Montgomery on the Welsh borders. He founded the UK Institute of Rural Health and the Welsh Rural Postgraduate Unit in 1997 and was instrumental in creating the European Rural and Isolated Practitioners Association (EURIPA) and remained its president until 2012. John was one of the founding members of the WONCA Working Party on Rural Practice and took over as Chair in 2013 from Professor Ian Couper. He is currently the Senior Lecturer in Rural and Global Health at Keele Medical School in the UK. His passion for rural practice remains unabated and he believes that despite successes to date, there is much more to do to reduce rural inequalities and improve health outcomes of rural people around the world. He is determined to engage with young doctors and the Young Doctor Movements around the world during his time as Chair. He believes strongly that the future of rural practice lies in their hands and the profession needs to engage and enthuse future rural doctors.

References[*]

Aaraas I J, Halvorsen P A. (2014) Developing rural medical schools: The history of Tromsø and Northern Norway. In Chater A B, Rourke J, Couper I D *et al.* (eds) *WONCA Rural Medical Education Guidebook*. Bangkok: WONCA Working Party on Rural Practice, World Organization of Family Doctors (WONCA), online at www.globalfamilyldoctor.com (accessed 16 March 2016).

Aaraas I J, Halvorsen P A, Aasland O G. (2015) Supply of doctors to a rural region: Occupations of Tromsø medical graduates 1979–2012. *Medical Teacher* **37:** 1078–82.

Aaraas I, Langfeldt E, Ersdal G *et al.* (2000) [The cottage hospital model, a key to better cooperation in health care – let the cottage hospital survive!]. *Tidsskrift for den Norske lægeforening* **120:** 702–5. [Article in Norwegian]

Akinkugbe O O. (2010) *Footprints & Footnotes: An autobiography*. Bookcraft: Ibadan.

Anon. (1984) Richard Scott. *Lancet* **323:** 58–9.

Arendt J. (2010) Shift work: coping with the biological clock. *Occupational Medicine* **60:** 10–20.

Asthana S, Halliday J, Gibson A. (2009) Social exclusion and social justice: a rural perspective on resource allocation. *Policy and Politics* **37:** 201–14.

Baird G, Hogg D. (2010) The RCGP's Rural Forum. *British Journal of General Practice* **60:** 295.

Baird A G, Jewell D, Walker J J. (1996) Management of labour in an isolated rural maternity hospital. *BMJ* **312:** 223–6.

Baird A G, Gillies J C, Bone F J *et al.* (1989) Prevalence of antibody indicating Lyme disease in farmers in Wigtownshire. *BMJ* **299:** 836–7.

Baird G, Flynn R, Baxter G *et al.* (2008) Travel time and cancer care: an example of the inverse care law? *Rural and Remote Health* **8:** 1003.

---

* Please note that references with four or more authors are cited using the first three names followed by 'et al.'. References with 'et al.' are organized in chronological order, not by second author, so as to be easily identifiable from the footnotes.

Bartlett M, McKinley R K, Wynn Jones J *et al.* (2011) A rural undergraduate campus in England: virtue from opportunity and necessity. *Rural Remote Health* (Internet) **11**: 1841, online at: www.rrh.org.au/articles/subviewnew. asp?ArticleID=1841 (accessed 28 June 2016).

Bellerose G. (2006) *Caring for Our Own: A portrait of community health care.* Middlebury, Vermont: Painter House Press.

Boelen C, Heck J. (1995) *Defining and Measuring the Social Accountability of Medical Schools.* Geneva: World Health Organization. (Unpublished document WHO/HRH/95.7, online at: http://apps.who.int/iris/ bitstream/10665/59441/1/WHO_HRH_95.7.pdf (accessed 28 June 2016).

Boelen C, Woollard B. (2009) Social accountability and accreditation: a new frontier for educational institutions. *Medical Education* **43**: 887–94.

Boelen C, Dharamsi S, Gibbs T. (2012) The social accountability of medical schools and its indicators. *Education for Health* **25**: 180–94.

Bourke S, Baird A G, Bone F J *et al.* (1988) Lyme disease with acute purulent meningitis. *British Medical Journal* **297**: 460.

British Medical Association. (1950) *General Practice and the Training of the General Practitioner: The report of a committee of the Association.* (Chaired by Henry Cohen) London: British Medical Association.

British Medical Association. (1965) *Charter for the Family Doctor Service.* London: British Medical Association.

British Medical Association, Board of Science. (2005) *Healthcare in a Rural Setting.* London: British Medical Association; available online at: http:// www.nsdm.no/filarkiv/File/Eksterne_rapporter/BMA.pdf (accessed 10 May 2016).

Buquet-Marcon C, Charlier P, Samzun A. (2007) The oldest amputation on a Neolithic human skeleton in France. *Nature Precedings.* Available at: http:// precedings.nature.com/documents/1278/version/1 (accessed 10 May 2016).

Cameron E A, Tindley A. (2015) *Dr Lachlan Grant of Ballachulish, 1871–1945.* Edinburgh: John Donald Publishers.

Campbell M. (1962) Paul Wood. *British Heart Journal* **24**: 661–6.

Chater B. (1993) The role of the National Rural Health Alliance. *Australian Journal of Rural Health* **1:** 5–12.

Chouinard J. (1983) Satellite contributions to telemedicine: Canadian CME experiences. *Canadian Medical Association Journal* **128:** 850–5.

Clough R. (ed.) (2012) *From a Broom Cupboard: 20 years of rural health at Monash University.* Melbourne: Monash University Publishing, available online at: http://books.publishing.monash.edu/apps/bookworm/view/From+a+broom+cupboard%3A+20+years+of+health+at+Monash+University/168/fbc-epub.html (accessed 10 May 2016).

Committee on Scottish Health Services. (1936) *Report of Committee on Scottish Health Services.* Chaired by Edward Cathcart. Edinburgh: HMSO (Cmd: 5204).

Commonwealth Department of Human Services and Health. (1994) *Rural Doctors: Reforming undergraduate medical education for rural practice. Final report of the Rural Undergraduate Steering Committee.* Canberra: Australian Government Publishing Service.

Couper I, Strasser R, Rourke J *et al.* (2015) Rural health activism over two decades: the WONCA Working Party on Rural Practice 1992–2012. *Rural and Remote Health* **15:** 3245, available online at www.rrh.org.au/publishedarticles/article_print_3245.pdf (accessed 15 March 2016).

Cox J. (ed.) (1995) *Rural General Practice in the UK,* occasional paper series no. 71. London: Royal College of General Practitioners.

Cox J, Mungall I. (eds) (1998) *Rural Healthcare.* CRC Press.

Curran V, Rourke J. (2004) The role of medical education in the recruitment and retention of rural physicians. *Medical Teacher* **26:** 265–72.

Department of Health. (2003) *Investing in General Practice: The new GMS contract.* London: Department of Health.

Department of the Environment, Transport and the Regions. (2000) *Our Countryside: The future – a fair deal for rural England.* London: The Stationery Office, online at: http://webarchive.nationalarchives.gov.uk/20050301192907/http://defra.gov.uk/rural/ruralwp/whitepaper/default.htm (accessed 12 April 2016).

Dixon J, Glennerster H. (1995) What do we know about fundholding in general practice? *BMJ* **311:** 727.

Doherty J, Conco D, Couper I *et al.* (2013) Developing a new mid-level health worker: lessons from South Africa's experience with clinical associates. *Global Health Action* **6:** 19282. doi: 10.3402/gha.v6i0.19282.

Donovan R, Bain J. (eds) (2000) *Single-handed: General practitioners in remote and rural areas.* Latheronwheel: Whittles.

Douglas J D. (1985) Medical problems of sport diving. *British Medical Journal (Clinical Research Edition)* **291:** 1224–6.

Douglas J D M. (2009) John A J MacLeod. *BMJ* **339:** b4296. doi: http://dx.doi.org/10.1136/bmj.b4296.

Douglas J D, Milne A H. (1991) Decompression sickness in fish farm workers: a new occupational hazard. *BMJ* **302:** 1244–5.

Douglas J, Tindley A, Smyth A. (2015) Dr Lachlan Grant (1871–1945). *Occupational Medicine* **64:** 233–4.

Douglas J D, McSharry C, Blaikie L *et al.* (1995) Occupational asthma caused by automated salmon processing. *Lancet* **346:** 737–40.

Duffy T P. (2011) The Flexner Report – 100 years later. *Yale Journal of Biology and Medicine* **84:** 269–76.

Elford R. (2009) Telemedicine activities at Memorial University of Newfoundland: a historical review, 1975–1997. *Telemedicine Journal* **4:** 207–24.

Flaherty J. (1998) Apprentices sample life of doctors in villages. *New York Times,* March 11, online at www.nytimes.com/1998/03/11/us/apprentices-sample-life-of-doctors-in-villages.html (accessed 29 June 2016).

Flexner A. (1910) *Medical Education in the United States and Canada. A Report to the Carnegie Foundation for the Advancement of Teaching.* New York: Carnegie Foundation for the Advancement of Teaching, Bulletin no. 4.

Freeman K, Wynn-Jones J, Groves-Phillips S *et al.* (1996) Teleconsulting: a practical account of pitfalls, problems and promise. Experience from the TEAM project group. *Journal of Telemedicine and Telecare* **2 (Suppl 1):** 1–3.

Gamnes J, Rasmussen K. (eds) (2013) *Fra Fagomradet medisin til Det helsevitenskapelige fakultet. Det medisinske fakultets historie, Universitetet i Tromsø* [The history of the medical faculty in Tromsø]. Orkana forlag [in Norwegian].

Gillies J C, Baird A G, Gillies E M. (1995) Balancing proactive and reactive care. *Occasional Paper (Royal College of General Practitioners)* **71:** 15–18.

Gill P, Wright N, Brew I. (eds) (2014) *Working with Vulnerable Groups: A clinical handbook for GPs.* London: RCGP.

Gordon I. (1989) Streptokinase used in general practice. *Journal of the Royal College of General Practitioners* **39:** 49–51.

Green L A, Fryer G E Jr, Yawn B P *et al.* (2001) The ecology of medical care revisited. *New England Journal of Medicine* **344:** 2021–25.

Greer S L. (2008) Devolution and divergence in UK health policies. *BMJ* **337:** doi: http://dx.doi.org/10.1136/bmj.a2616 (accessed 10 May 2016).

Grol R, Giesen P, van Uden C. (2006) After-hours care in the United Kingdom, Denmark, and the Netherlands: new models. *Health Affairs* **25:** 1733–7.

Hallam L. (1994) Primary medical care outside normal working hours: review of published work. *BMJ* **308:** 249–53.

Hamilton J. (2011) The renewal of medical education in Iran: progress and challenge. *Medical Journal of Islamic Republic of Iran* **25:** 53–6.

Hammett D. (2007) Cuban intervention in South African health care service provision. *Journal of Southern African Studies* **33:** 63–81.

Hays R. (2001) Rural initiatives at the James Cook University School of Medicine: a vertically integrated regional/rural/remote medical education provider. *Australian Journal of Rural Health* **9:** S2–5.

Hays R. (2002) *Practising Rural Medicine in Australia.* Emerald, Victoria: Eruditions Publishing.

Hays R B. (2003a) Ruralising medical education curricula: the importance of context in problem design. *Australian Journal of Rural Health* **11:** 15–17.

Hays R B. (2003b) Rural medical education: how different is it? *Medical Education* **37:** 4–5.

Hays R B. (2007) Interprofessional education in the community: where to begin. *The Clinical Teacher* **4:** 141–5.

Hays R B. (2008) Interprofessional education in rural practice: how, when and where? *Rural and Remote Health* **8:** 939.

Hays R. (2014) Developing a rural medical school in Australia. Chapter 2.1.7 WONCA Rural Medical Education Guidebook, online at www.globalfamilydoctor.com/groups/WorkingParties/RuralPractice/ruralguidebook.aspx (accessed 31 May 2016).

Hays R B, Bower A. (2001) Modifying academic ranking of rural and remote medical school applicants. *Medical Journal of Australia* **174:** 371–2.

Hays R B, Stokes J, Veitch J. (2003) A new socially responsible medical school for regional Australia. *Education for Health* **16:** 14–21.

Hays R B, Veitch J, Lam A. (2005) Teaching clinical pathology by flexible delivery in rural sites. *Australian Journal of Rural Health* **13:** 232–5.

Hays R B, Veitch P C, Cheers B *et al.* (1997) Why doctors leave rural practice. *Australian Journal of Rural Health* **5:** 198–203.

Hudson G, Hunt D. (2009) Social Accountability and the Northern Ontario School of Medicine. In Tesson G, Hudson G, Strasser R *et al.* (eds) (2009) *The Making of the Northern Ontario School of Medicine: A case history in the history of medical education.* Montreal/Kingston: McGill-Queen's University Press, 157–82

Hudson G, Maar M. (2014) Faculty analysis of distributed medical education in Northern Canadian Aboriginal communities. *Rural and Remote Health.* **14:** 2664.

Humber N, Frecker T. (2008) Delivery models of rural surgical services in British Columbia (1996–2005): are general practitioner–surgeons still part of the picture? *Canadian Journal of Surgery* **51:** 173–8.

Jarman B. (1983) Identification of underprivileged areas. *BMJ* (Clinical Research Edition) **286:** 1705–9.

Jensen E B. (2008) *Fra krisetiltak til suksesshistorier. Desentraliserte profesjonsutdanninger i Troms 1978–2008* [From crisis intervention to success stories. Decentralised professional educations in Troms 1978–2008]. Orkana forlag [in Norwegian].

Kaufman A, Powell W, Alfero C *et al.* (2010) Health extension in New Mexico: an academic health center and the social determinants of disease. *Annals of Family Medicine* **8:** 73–81.

Kay A. (2002) The abolition of the GP fundholding scheme: a lesson in evidence-based policy making. *British Journal of General Practice* **52:** 141–4.

Kermode-Scott B. (2012) Ian Renwick McWhinney *BMJ* **345:** e7450.

Lehmann U. (2008) *Mid-level Health Workers: The state of the evidence on programmes, activities, costs and impact on health outcomes; A literature review.* Geneva: World Health Organization; 2008. Available online at www.who. int/hrh/MLHW_review_2008.pdf (accessed 31 May 2016).

Leng T P. (2011) *An Uncommon Hero: M K Rajakumar in politics and medicine.* Petaling Jaya: Strategic Information and Research Development Centre.

MacVicar R, Clarke G, Hogg D R. (2016) Scotland's GP Rural Fellowship: an initiative that has impacted on rural recruitment and retention. *Rural and Remote Health* **16:** 3550, available online at www.rrh.org.au/articles/ subviewnew.asp?ArticleID=3550 (accessed 27 July 2016).

Marmot M. (2010) *Fair Society, Healthy Lives: The Marmot Review: strategic review of health inequalities in England post-2010,* online at www. instituteofhealthequity.org/projects/fair-society-healthy-lives-the-marmot-review (accessed 4 October 2016).

Marshall L. (1997) Associate general practitioners. *BMJ* **315:** S2–7102.

Mather H G, Morgan D V, Pearson N G *et al.* (1976) Myocardial infarction: a comparison between home and hospital care for patients. *BMJ* **i:** 925–9.

Maudsley R F, Wilson D R, Neufeld V R *et al.* (2000) Educating future physicians for Ontario: phase II. *Academic Medicine* **75:** 113–26.

Meslin E M. (1987) The moral costs of the Ontario physicians' strike. *The Hastings Center Report* **17:** 11–14.

Miflin B, Price D. (1993) Rural doctors are naturally effective teachers. *Australian Journal of Rural Health* **2:** 21–8, doi: 10.1111/j.1440-1584.1993. tb00094.x.

Monash University Centre for Rural Health, University of Queensland Northern Queensland Clinical School, Flinders University Rural & Remote Health Unit. (1998) *Development of Models for Sustainable General Practice Services in Rural and Remote Areas.* Canberra: DH&FS.

Murray R B, Larkins L, Russell H *et al.* (2012) Medical schools as agents of change: socially accountable medical education. *Medical Journal of Australia* **196:** 653, doi: 10.5694/mja11.11473.

Ness A R, Reynolds L A, Tansey E M. (eds) (2002) *Population-based Research in South Wales: The MRC Pneumoconiosis Research Unit and the MRC Epidemiology Unit.* Wellcome Witnesses to Twentieth Century Medicine, vol. 13. London: The Wellcome Trust Centre for the History of Medicine at UCL; available online at www.histmodbiomed.org/witsem/vol13 (accessed 10 October 2016).

Neufeld V R, Maudsley R F, Pickering R J *et al.* (1998) Educating future physicians for Ontario. *Academic Medicine* **73:** 1133–48.

Nichols A, Streeton M-J, Cowie M. (2002) Australian College of Rural and Remote Medicine. *Australian Journal of Rural Health* **10:** 263–4.

Overy C, Tansey E M. (eds) (2014) *The Recent History of Seasonal Affective Disorder (SAD).* Wellcome Witnesses to Contemporary Medicine, vol. 51. London: Queen Mary University of London, available online at: www. histmodbiomed.org/witsem/vol51 (accessed 23 May 2016).

Parry E H O. (ed.) (1976) *Principles of Medicine in Africa.* Oxford: Oxford University Press.

Parry E H O, Ikeme A C. (1966) *Cardiovascular Disease in Nigeria.* Ibadan: Department of Medicine, University College Hospital, Ibadan University.

Peckham S. (2007) The new General Practice contract and reform of primary care in the United Kingdom. *Healthcare Policy* **2:** 34–48.

Pemberton J. (1969) William Pickles. *British Journal of General Practice* **18:** 5–8.

Pickles W N. (1939) *Epidemiology in a Country Practice.* (Bristol: J Wright); republished (1972) Exeter: Royal College of General Practitioners.

Račić: M. (2015) Family medicine development in Bosnia and Herzegovina. *Journal of Family Medicine* **2:** 1031, online at http://austinpublishinggroup.com/family-medicine/fulltext/jfm-v2-id1031.php (accessed 31 May 2016).

Reynolds L A, Tansey E M. (1998) Research in general practice. In Tansey E M, Christie D A, Reynolds L A. (eds) (1998) *Wellcome Witnesses to Twentieth Century Medicine*, vol. 2. London: The Wellcome Trust, 75–130; available online at www.histmodbiomed.org/witsem/vol2 (accessed 10 October 2016).

Reynolds L A, Tansey E M. (eds) (2003) *Foot and Mouth Disease: The 1967 outbreak and its aftermath.* Wellcome Witnesses to Twentieth Century Medicine, vol. 18. London: Wellcome Trust Centre for the History of Medicine at UCL; available online at: www.histmodbiomed.org/witsem/vol18 (accessed 29 June 2016).

Reynolds L A, Tansey E M. (eds) (2008) *Clinical Pharmacology in the UK, c.1950–2000: Influences and institutions.* Wellcome Witnesses to Twentieth Century Medicine, vol. 33. London: The Wellcome Trust Centre for the History of Medicine at UCL; available online at www.histmodbiomed.org/witsem/vol33 (accessed 10 October 2016).

Ross S J, Preston R, Lindemann I *et al.* (2014) The training for health equity network evaluation framework: a pilot study at five health professional schools. *Education for Health* **27:** 116–26.

Rourke J T B, Incitti F, Rourke L L *et al.* (2003) Keeping family physicians in rural practice. Solutions favoured by rural physicians and family medicine residents. *Canadian Family Physician* **49:** 1142–9.

Sackett D L, Rosenberg W M C, Gray J A M *et al.* (1996) Evidence based medicine: what it is and what it isn't. *BMJ* **312:** 71–2, doi: http://dx.doi.org/10.1136/bmj.312.7023.71 (accessed 16 March 2016).

Sage A. (2010) Evidence of Stone Age amputation forces rethink over history of surgery. *The Times* (25 January).

Schmidt H G, Neufeld V R, Nooman Z M *et al.* (1991) Network of community oriented educational institutions for the health sciences. *Academic Medicine* **66:** 259–63.

Schön D. (1967) *Technology and Change: The new Heraclitus.* New York: Delacorte Press.

Schön D. (1971) *Beyond the Stable State. Public and private learning in a changing society.* London: Maurice Temple Smith.

Schön D. (1983) *The Reflective Practitioner. How professionals think in action.* London: Temple Smith.

Scott B. (2013) Arthur Maxwell House. *BMJ* **347:** doi: http://dx.doi.org/10.1136/bmj.f7188 (accessed 10 October 2016).

Scottish Office. (1998) *Acute Services Review* (Carter Report). Edinburgh: Scottish Office Publications.

Sen Gupta T K, Murray R B, McDonell A *et al.* (2008) Rural internships for final year students: clinical experience, education and workforce. *Rural and Remote Health* **8:** 827, available online at www.rrh.org.au/articles/subviewnew.asp?ArticleID=827 (accessed 10 October 2016).

Sen Gupta T, Woolley T, Murray R *et al.* (2014) Positive impacts on rural and regional workforce from the first seven cohorts of James Cook University medical graduates. *Rural and Remote Health* **14:** 2657, available online at www.rrh.org.au/articles/subviewnew.asp?ArticleID=2657 (accessed 10 October 2016).

Smith J D, Hays R B. (2004) Is rural medical practice a separate discipline? *Australian Journal of Rural Health* **12:** 67–72.

Smith R. (2015) David Sackett. *BMJ* **350:** doi: http://dx.doi.org/10.1136/bmj.h2639 (accessed 16 March 2016).

Spaulding W B. (1969) The undergraduate medical curriculum (1969 model): McMaster University. *Canadian Medical Association Journal* **100:** 659–64.

Spaulding W B. (1991) *Revitalizing Medical Education: McMaster Medical School, the early years, 1965–74.* Philadelphia, PA: B C Decker Inc.

Starfield B, Shi L, Macinko J. (2005) Contribution of primary care to health systems and health. *Milbank Quarterly* **83:** 457–502.

Steedman D J, Gordon M W G, Cusack S *et al.* (1991) Lessons for mobile medical teams following the Lockerbie and Guthrie Street disasters. *Injury* **22:** 215–18.

Strasser R. (1995) Rural general practice: is it a distinct discipline? *Australian Family Physician* **24:** 870–1, 874–6.

Strasser R. (1997) From Shanghai to Durban: international rural health conferences. *Australian Journal of Rural Health* **5:** 165–8.

Strasser R. (2016) Delivering on social accountability: Canada's Northern Ontario School of Medicine. *The Asia Pacific Scholar* **1:** 3–9.

Strasser R, Neusy A-J. (2010) Context counts: training health workers in and for rural and remote areas. *Bulletin of the World Health Organization* **88:** 777–82.

Strasser R, Kam S M, Regalado S M. (2016) Rural health care access and policy in developing countries. *Annual Review of Public Health* **37:** 395–412.

Strasser R P, Lanphear J H, McCready W G *et al.* (2009) Canada's new medical school: The Northern Ontario School of Medicine: social accountability through distributed community engaged learning. *Academic Medicine* **84:** 1459–64.

Strasser R, Hogenbirk J C, Minore B *et al.* (2013) Transforming health professional education through social accountability: Canada's Northern Ontario School of Medicine. *Medical Teacher* **35:** 490–6.

Strasser R, Couper I, Wynn-Jones J *et al.* (2016) Education for rural practice in rural practice. *Education for Primary Care* **27:** 10–14.

Strasser S, Strasser R P. (2007) The Northern Ontario School of Medicine: a long-term strategy to enhance the rural medical workforce. *Cahiers de Sociologie et de Démographie Médicales* **47:** 469–89.

Swindlehurst H F, Deaville J A, Wynn-Jones J *et al.* (2005) Rural proofing for health: a commentary. *Rural and Remote Health* (Internet) **5:** 411, available online at www.rrh.org.au/articles/subviewnew.asp?ArticleID=411 (accessed 31 May 2016).

Tesson G, Hudson G, Strasser R *et al.* (eds) (2009) *The Making of the Northern Ontario School of Medicine: A case study in the history of medical education.* Montreal/Kingston: McGill-Queen's University Press.

Tollman S M (1994) The Pholela Health Centre – The origins of community-oriented primary health care (COPC). An appreciation of the work of Sidney and Emily Kark. *South African Medical Journal* **84:** 653–8.

Tooke J. (2008) *Aspiring to Excellence: Findings and recommendations of the Independent Inquiry into Modernising Medical Careers.* London: MMC Inquiry.

UK Health Departments. (2004) *Modernising Medical Careers. The next steps. The future shape of Foundation, Specialist and General Practice Training Programmes.* Department of Health, online at: http://webarchive.nationalarchives.gov.uk/20130107105354/http:/dh.gov.uk/prod_consum_dh/groups/dh_digitalassets/@dh/@en/documents/digitalasset/dh_4079532.pdf (accessed 27 June 2016).

Veitch C, Underhill A, Hays R B. (2006) The career aspirations and location intentions of James Cook University's first cohort of medical students: a longitudinal study at course entry and graduation. *Rural and Remote Health* **6:** 537, available online at www.rrh.org.au/articles/subviewnew.asp?ArticleID=537 (accessed 10 October 2016).

Verby J E. (1988) The Minnesota Rural Physician Associate Program for medical students. *Journal of Medical Education.* **63:** 427–37.

Walpole R. (1979) *Rural Health, Proceedings of the Rural Health Conference of RACGP.* Melbourne: Newtone Press.

Wearne S, Giddings P, McLaren J *et al.* (2010) Where are they now? The career paths of the Remote Vocational Training Scheme registrars. *Australian Family Physician* **39:** 53–6.

Wibulpolprasert S, Pengpaiboon P. (2003) Integrated strategies to tackle the inequitable distribution of doctors in Thailand: four decades of experience. *Human Resources for Health* **1:** 12, doi: 10.1186/1478-4491-1-12.

Wilkinson D, Laven G, Pratt N *et al.* (2003) Impact of undergraduate and postgraduate rural training, and medical school entry criteria on rural practice among Australian general practitioners: national study of 2414 doctors. *Medical Education* **37:** 809–14.

WONCA (1998) *Using Information Technology to Improve Rural Healthcare.* World Organization of Family Doctors, available online at www.globalfamilydoctor.com/site/DefaultSite/filesystem/documents/Groups/Rural%20Practice/information%20technology%20rural%20health%201998.PDF (accessed 10 October 2016).

WONCA Working Party on Rural Practice. (1995) *Policy on Training for Rural General Practice*, available online at www.globalfamilydoctor.com/groups/WorkingParties/RuralPractice.aspx (accessed 31 May 2016).

WONCA Working Party on Rural Practice. (2003) *Policy on Female Family Physicians in Rural Practice.* 2nd ed. Traralgon, Vic: Monash University School of Rural Health.

Woollard R F. (2006) Caring for a common future: medical schools' social accountability. *Medical Education* **40**: 301–13.

Woolley T, Sen Gupta T, Murray R *et al.* (2014) Predictors of rural practice location for James Cook University MBBS graduates at postgraduate year 5. *Australian Journal of Rural Health* **22**: 165–71.

World Health Organization. (2010) *Increasing Access to Health Workers in Remote and Rural Areas through Improved Retention. Global policy recommendations.* Geneva: World Health Organization; available online at: www.who.int/hrh/retention/guidelines/en/ (accessed 17 October 2016).

World Health Organization. (2013) *Transforming and Scaling up Health Professionals' Education and Training: World Health Organization guidelines in 2013.* Geneva: World Health Organization; available online at www.who.int/hrh/resources/transf_scaling_hpet/en/ (accessed 13 April 2016).

World Health Organization/WONCA. (1995) *Making Medical Practice and Education more Relevant to People's Needs: The contribution of the family doctor.* Working Paper. Geneva: World Health Organization. The Working party report is available online at http://apps.who.int/iris/bitstream/10665/62364/1/55633.pdf (accessed 20 April 2016).

Worley P S, Prideaux D J, Strasser R P *et al.* (2000) Why we should teach undergraduate medical students in rural communities. *Medical Journal of Australia* **172**: 615–17.

Index: Subject

Page numbers in *italics* refer to illustrations.

Index: Names

Page numbers in *italics* refer to photographs,
those in **bold** refer to biographical notes.

VOLUMES IN THIS SERIES*

1. **Technology transfer in Britain: The case of monoclonal antibodies**
   Self and non-self: A history of autoimmunity
   Endogenous opiates
   The Committee on Safety of Drugs (1997) ISBN 1 86983 579 4

2. **Making the human body transparent: The impact of NMR and MRI**
   Research in general practice
   Drugs in psychiatric practice
   The MRC Common Cold Unit (1998) ISBN 1 86983 539 5

3. **Early heart transplant surgery in the UK (1999)** ISBN 1 84129 007 6

4. **Haemophilia: Recent history of clinical management (1999)**
   ISBN 1 84129 008 4

5. **Looking at the unborn: Historical aspects of**
   obstetric ultrasound (2000) ISBN 1 84129 011 4

6. **Post penicillin antibiotics: From acceptance to resistance? (2000)**
   ISBN 1 84129 012 2

7. **Clinical research in Britain, 1950–1980 (2000)**
   ISBN 1 84129 016 5

8. **Intestinal absorption (2000)**
   ISBN 1 84129 017 3

9. **Neonatal intensive care (2001)**
   ISBN 0 85484 076 1

10. **British contributions to medical research and education in Africa**
    after the Second World War (2001) ISBN 0 85484 077 X

* All volumes are freely available online at: www.histmodbiomed.org/article/wellcome-witnesses-volumes .They can also be purchased from www.amazon.co.uk; www.amazon.com, and from all good booksellers.

11. **Childhood asthma and beyond (2001)**
ISBN 0 85484 078 8

12. **Maternal care (2001)**
ISBN 0 85484 079 6

13. **Population-based research in south Wales: The MRC Pneumoconiosis Research Unit and the MRC Epidemiology Unit (2002)**
ISBN 0 85484 081 8

14. **Peptic ulcer: Rise and fall (2002)**
ISBN 0 85484 084 2

15. **Leukaemia (2003)**
ISBN 0 85484 087 7

16. **The MRC Applied Psychology Unit (2003)**
ISBN 0 85484 088 5

17. **Genetic testing (2003)**
ISBN 0 85484 094 X

18. **Foot and mouth disease: The 1967 outbreak and its aftermath (2003)**
ISBN 0 85484 096 6

19. **Environmental toxicology: The legacy of *Silent Spring* (2004)**
ISBN 0 85484 091 5

20. **Cystic fibrosis (2004)**
ISBN 0 85484 086 9

21. **Innovation in pain management (2004)**
ISBN 978 0 85484 097 7

22. **The Rhesus factor and disease prevention (2004)**
ISBN 978 0 85484 099 1

23. **The recent history of platelets in thrombosis and other disorders (2005)** ISBN 978 0 85484 103 5

24. **Short-course chemotherapy for tuberculosis (2005)**
ISBN 978 0 85484 104 2

25. **Prenatal corticosteroids for reducing morbidity and mortality after preterm birth (2005)** ISBN 978 0 85484 102 8

26. **Public health in the 1980s and 1990s: Decline and rise? (2006)**
ISBN 978 0 85484 106 6

27. **Cholesterol, atherosclerosis and coronary disease in the UK, 1950–2000 (2006)** ISBN 978 0 85484 107 3

28. **Development of physics applied to medicine in the UK, 1945–1990 (2006)** ISBN 978 0 85484 108 0

29. **Early development of total hip replacement (2007)**
ISBN 978 0 85484 111 0

30. **The discovery, use and impact of platinum salts as chemotherapy agents for cancer (2007)** ISBN 978 0 85484 112 7

31. **Medical ethics education in Britain, 1963–1993 (2007)**
ISBN 978 0 85484 113 4

32. **Superbugs and superdrugs: A history of MRSA (2008)**
ISBN 978 0 85484 114 1

33. **Clinical pharmacology in the UK, _c._ 1950–2000: Influences and institutions (2008)** ISBN 978 0 85484 117 2

34. **Clinical pharmacology in the UK, _c._ 1950–2000: Industry and regulation (2008)** ISBN 978 0 85484 118 9

35. **The resurgence of breastfeeding, 1975–2000 (2009)**
ISBN 978 0 85484 119 6

36. **The development of sports medicine in twentieth-century Britain (2009)** ISBN 978 0 85484 121 9

37. **History of dialysis, *c.*1950–1980 (2009)** ISBN 978 0 85484 122 6

38. **History of cervical cancer and the role of the human papillomavirus, 1960–2000 (2009)** ISBN 978 0 85484 123 3

39. **Clinical genetics in Britain: Origins and development (2010)** ISBN 978 0 85484 127 1

40. **The medicalization of cannabis (2010)** ISBN 978 0 85484 129 5

41. **History of the National Survey of Sexual Attitudes and Lifestyles (2011)** ISBN 978 0 90223 874 9

42. **History of British intensive care, *c.*1950–*c.*2000 (2011)** ISBN 978 0 90223 875 6

43. **WHO Framework Convention on Tobacco Control (2012)** ISBN 978 0 90223 877 0

44. **History of the Avon Longitudinal Study of Parents and Children (ALSPAC), *c.*1980–2000 (2012)** ISBN 978 0 90223 878 7

45. **Palliative medicine in the UK *c.*1970–2010 (2013)** ISBN 978 0 90223 882 4

46. **Clinical cancer genetics: Polyposis and familial colorectal cancer *c.*1975–*c.*2010 (2013)** ISBN 978 0 90223 885 5

47. **Drugs affecting 5-HT systems (2013)** ISBN 978 0 90223 887 9

48. **Clinical molecular genetics in the UK *c.*1975–*c.*2000 (2014)** ISBN 978 0 90223 888 6

49. **Migraine: Diagnosis, treatment and understanding *c.*1960–2010 (2014)** ISBN 978 0 90223 894 7

50. **Monoclonal antibodies to migraine: Witnesses to modern biomedicine, an A–Z (2014)** ISBN 978 0 90223 895 4

51. **The recent history of seasonal affective disorder (SAD) (2014)**
ISBN 978 0 90223 897 8

52. **The development of narrative practices in medicine *c.*1960–*c.*2000 (2015)** ISBN 978 0 90223 898 5

53. **The development of brain banks in the UK *c.*1970–*c.*2010 (2015)**
ISBN 978 1 91019 5024

54. **Human Gene Mapping Workshops *c.*1973–*c.*1991 (2015)**
ISBN 978 1 91019 5031

55. **A history of bovine TB *c.*1965–*c.*2000 (2015)**
ISBN 978 1 91019 5055

56. **The development of waste management in the UK *c.*1960–*c.*2000 (2015)** ISBN 978 1 91019 5062

57. **Medical genetics: Development of ethical dimensions in clinical practice and research (2016)** ISBN 978 1 91019 5130

58. **Air pollution research in Britain *c.*1955–*c.*2000 (2016)**
ISBN 978 1 91019 5147

59. **Technology, techniques, and technicians at the National Institute for Medical Research (NIMR) *c.*1960–*c.*2000 (2016)**
ISBN 978 1 91019 5161

60. **The recent history of tumour necrosis factor (TNF) (2016)**
ISBN 978 1 91019 5208

61. **Historical perspectives on rural medicine. The proceedings of two Witness Seminars (2017)**
ISBN 978 1 91019 5222 (this volume)

UNPUBLISHED WITNESS SEMINARS

1994	**The early history of renal transplantation**

1994 Pneumoconiosis of coal workers
(partially published in volume 13, *Population-based research in south Wales*)

1995 Oral contraceptives

2003 Beyond the asylum: Anti-psychiatry and care in the community

2003 Thrombolysis
(partially published in volume 27, *Cholesterol, atherosclerosis and coronary disease in the UK, 1950–2000*)

2007 DNA fingerprinting

The transcripts and records of all Witness Seminars are held in archives and manuscripts, Wellcome Library, London, at GC/253.

OTHER PUBLICATIONS

Technology transfer in Britain: The case of monoclonal antibodies
Tansey E M, Catterall P P. (1993) *Contemporary Record* **9**: 409–44.

Monoclonal antibodies: A witness seminar on contemporary medical history
Tansey E M, Catterall P P. (1994) *Medical History* **38**: 322–7.

Chronic pulmonary disease in South Wales coalmines: An eye-witness account of the MRC surveys (1937–42)
P D'Arcy Hart, edited and annotated by E M Tansey. (1998)
Social History of Medicine **11**: 459–68.

Ashes to Ashes – The history of smoking and health
Lock S P, Reynolds L A, Tansey E M. (eds) (1998) Amsterdam: Rodopi BV,
228pp. ISBN 90420 0396 0 (Hfl 125) (hardback). Reprinted 2003.

Witnessing medical history. An interview with Dr Rosemary Biggs
Professor Christine Lee and Dr Charles Rizza (interviewers). (1998)
Haemophilia **4**: 769–77.

Witnessing the Witnesses: Pitfalls and potentials of the Witness Seminar in twentieth century medicine
Tansey E M, in Doel R, Søderqvist T. (eds) (2006) *Writing Recent Science: The historiography of contemporary science, technology and medicine.* London: Routledge: 260–78.

The Witness Seminar technique in modern medical history
Tansey E M, in Cook H J, Bhattacharya S, Hardy A. (eds) (2008) *History of the Social Determinants of Health: Global Histories, Contemporary Debates.* London: Orient Longman: 279–95.

Today's medicine, tomorrow's medical history
Tansey E M, in Natvig J B, Swärd E T, Hem E. (eds) (2009) *Historier om helse* (*Histories about Health,* in Norwegian). Oslo: *Journal of the Norwegian Medical Association:* 166–73.

Key to cover photographs

Front cover, left to right
Professor Roger Strasser
Professor James Rourke
Professor Richard Hays
Professor Sarah Strasser
Dr James Douglas

Back cover, left to right
Professor John Hamilton
Professor Bruce Chater
Professor Ian Couper
Dr John Wynn-Jones
Professor Ivar Aaraas

Lightning Source UK Ltd.
Milton Keynes UK
UKOW07f2030280217
295582UK00001B/74/P